STRENGTHS IN
THE MIRROR

STRENGTHS IN THE MIRROR

THRIVING NOW AND TOMORROW

LIANA LIANOV, MD, MPH

NDP

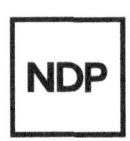

NEW DEGREE PRESS
COPYRIGHT © 2021 LIANA LIANOV
All rights reserved.

STRENGTHS IN THE MIRROR
THRIVING NOW AND TOMORROW

ISBN   978-1-63676-787-1   *Paperback*
       978-1-63676-788-8   *Kindle Ebook*
       978-1-63676-789-5   *Ebook*

Few men during their lifetime come anywhere near exhausting the resources dwelling within them. There are deep wells of strength that are never used.

—RICHARD E. BYRD

While escaping from communist Bulgaria, my parents left all their family, their belongings, and their entire world to give me a better life and a hopeful future.

When I share the story of adopting my daughter, Lorelei, I often am told how lucky she is to have me as her mother. I reply that I am the lucky one, as her spirited, loving soul saved me. Across continents and oceans, a force brought us together to embrace life as a family.

I lovingly dedicate this book to Tania and Stefan Lianov and Lorelei Bergerson.

CONTENTS

PART 1.   LAYING THE GROUNDWORK   **1**

INTRODUCTION.   INSPIRATION AND DIRECTION   3

CHAPTER 1.   HOW DID WE GET HERE?   15

CHAPTER 2.   WHY NOW?   27

CHAPTER 3.   STRENGTHS WE CREATE   39

CHAPTER 4.   NATURAL STRENGTHS   53

PART 2.   RECOGNIZING OUR STRENGTHS   **69**

CHAPTER 5.   SELF-CARE STRENGTHS   71

CHAPTER 6.   POSITIVE ACTIVITY STRENGTHS   85

CHAPTER 7.   SOCIAL CONNECTION STRENGTHS   101

CHAPTER 8.   CHARACTER STRENGTHS   117

CHAPTER 9.   BRAIN STRENGTHS   129

PART 3.   APPLYING OUR STRENGTHS   **145**

CHAPTER 10. RELIABLE STRENGTHS DURING TRAUMA   147

CHAPTER 11. STRENGTHS IN ACTION   159

EPILOGUE. THRIVING NOW AND TOMORROW   171

PART 4.   RESOURCES   **177**

IDENTIFYING BRAIN STRENGTHS   179

ADDITIONAL GUIDANCE AND TOOLS   187

ACKNOWLEDGMENTS   189

APPENDIX   193

PART 1

LAYING THE GROUNDWORK

INTRODUCTION

INSPIRATION AND DIRECTION

My Inspiration

I was born in Sofia, Bulgaria, behind the "Iron Curtain," during its communist times. Oppression was all around us; free expression was not allowed, and the government would often take away individual property to share with other citizens. We were moved from our comfortable apartment home to a cramped replacement, or outright evicted, more than once. This experience was unsettling and frightening for my parents. The government dictated how every citizen should live for the common good. There were no opportunities for the pursuit of individual endeavors nor for building personal passions. My parents eventually decided to escape when I was just five years old.

While my father was attending a medical conference in Vienna, Austria, he managed to convince the Bulgarian government that he had returned home. My mother and I were then allowed to vacation in neighboring Belgrade, Yugoslavia, which was still behind the Iron Curtain. We bought Yugoslavian passports from an undercover ring and boarded a train for Vienna.

At the border, my mother drugged me so that I would not give away the fact that we did not speak the native language. She also stuffed some cotton in her mouth and pretended to have a tooth infection. We successfully convinced the conductor that we were legitimate Yugoslavians who, at the time, could travel outside of communist borders. We reunited with my father in the free world and two years later arrived in Boston, Massachusetts. The US became my real home.

Despite this amazing achievement of giving his family a better life, my father spent the rest of his life unhappy, trying to fit into American culture and fulfill its expectations. Immediately upon arriving in the US, he insisted on taking English lessons and devoured the textbook in just a few weeks. This same determination helped him but also haunted him throughout his professional career, as he re-entered medical school to get trained and certified within the US medical system. The long hours and stress of keeping up alongside medical residents two decades younger led to his depression, overall poor health, then later cancer and death.

My father struggled to keep up according to his vision of what American life portrayed and his deep desire to fit into this new world, only to stir up deep unhappiness. He ignored his individuality, his culture, his health, and his family, working almost all the time. He started a medical practice without success due to language and cultural barriers. These struggles led to his death at a relatively young age, and he died a broken man. During one of our last conversations, he implored me, with authentic tears, not to follow his path but to do what makes me happy.

Pursuing a Career That Makes a Difference

With the memory of my father haunting me, it's no wonder I often questioned what constitutes a happy life and what I could do differently to avoid my father's fate. Better yet, how could I be prepared for life's inevitable challenges and grow through those experiences? What pillars could I rely on to thrive no matter what?

These questions lingered. In the ensuing years, I graduated from medical school, completed internal medicine and preventive medicine/public health residencies, and managed public health programs for the California Department of Health Services. Throughout this time, I was not satisfied with my work.

What could I offer professionally to help others achieve wellbeing? I spent much of my leisure time studying human behavior, what motivates us and what makes us truly happy and healthy. I took a leave of absence from my government position to complete a psychiatry fellowship and later decided to pursue a career in building educational programs that leverage the best scientific knowledge about health and happiness. I wanted to see how people can achieve these states despite human challenges and stressful situations.

Beyond Striving to Thriving and Antifragility

Can one navigate through the storms of life and come out the other end better than before? I say yes; that's thriving and antifragility. Thriving means more than successfully navigating difficult situations. It is the result of our growth when using our strengths on an ongoing basis to prepare physically, mentally, and emotionally for the full range of life experiences. Through a few essential habits, we can become our healthy, happy best selves, a version of ourselves ready to grow from anything we encounter. Many individuals struggle with everyday challenges like working long hours and occasional traumatic events like losing a loved one. They endure small and large arrows one after another and can't imagine they have the strengths to overcome difficulties, let alone be happy. Yet solutions are at their fingertips.

By building on our inner core, we cannot only cope, not only become resilient, but also flourish and even become, as discussed by Nassim Nicolas Taleb, antifragile (Taleb, 2020). Taleb says, "The resilient resists shocks and stays the same; the antifragile gets better." Being prepared for adversity and becoming antifragile often boils down to using our internal strengths and persisting with wellbeing activities that can be thought of as tools in our thriving toolkit.

Although several of my Author's Circle members prefer the term antifragile to thriving, I've chosen the latter because I want to avoid readers getting stuck on the "fragile" part of the word. Our brains tend to discount negative descriptors. When someone instructs you not to think of a white elephant, for example, your mind might be tempted to do the opposite! The term thriving (which I use interchangeably with flourishing) conjures a positive image and, here, I use it to mean enjoying excellent wellbeing across the core elements of health broadly defined—physical, mental, emotional, social, and spiritual. I also include "positive health," achieved by adopting mindsets and practices based on positive psychology. From this core, we can build success in other aspects of our lives, including professional and financial.

Recognizing Our Thriving Toolkit

The first step on the road to thriving is to recognize our strengths and the essential activities needed for thriving. What's in the toolkit? Physical health habits, positive activities, social support, character strengths, and brain strengths comprise the essential tools. In this book, we'll unpack these tools and view them through the lens and stories of respected colleagues.

Indeed, scientific and medical experts who have conducted research on mental and emotional wellbeing corroborate that advice. For example, Hendriks, a leading positive psychology researcher, analyzed a wide variety of studies on positive mindsets and activities, such as acts of kindness and forgiveness, and found something striking. Despite the diversity of these interventions, together, they indicate a statistically significant improvement in psychological wellbeing (Hendriks et al., 2019). Much more research is needed and is being conducted and published in the psychology and health journals to help refine these wellbeing approaches. In the meantime, we can take advantage of what is known.

Refining and Bolstering Our Thriving Toolkit

Building the right habits and self-confidence in our strengths takes effort and practice. Some of these strengths come to us naturally, while others need to be developed. Yet they all need to be used consistently. We cannot turn to them only as we face a crisis. Use the strength tools throughout life in order to sail through and grow in response to tough times.

How do we sharpen these tools? In addition to regular practice, the real trick is to build them in ways that ring true to our core selves. We must dig deep into what will truly work for each of us individually. We need to personalize our strength tools so that they feel comfortable and sustainable by aligning with our internal character strengths and our personality-based talents.

The guidance here is based on the fields of positive psychology, lifestyle medicine, and individual strengths. Together these approaches comprise the foundation of an approach that can keep us in a steady state of thriving. The five toolsets include:

1. Practicing healthy behaviors—We'll look at health behaviors with which you are likely already familiar—eating a predominantly whole-food, plant-based diet, being physically active, and getting enough quality sleep—through a new lens. How do these familiar habits relate to being happy, and how does being happy boost these behaviors?
2. Positive activities—You can build these activities into habits, like any healthy behavior. I'll make the case that a total healthy lifestyle should include these kinds of positive, intentional activities. This toolset also encompasses meaningful activities and approaches to a life with purpose, including spirituality and religion.
3. Social supports in your environment—The people we interact with positively on a daily or regular basis

personally and professionally represent the heart of this element.
4. Character strengths—Our highest character strengths, called signature strengths, can be identified by a scientifically validated questionnaire. We'll explore what these strengths are and learn from experts on how to best leverage them.
5. Brain strengths—We'll learn to identify and harness mental processes that come naturally to us and are aligned with our personalities. These eight mental processes were identified by the well-known psychiatrist Carl Jung and were used by Elizabeth Myers and Isabella Briggs to develop the Myers-Briggs Type Indicator of sixteen personality types. We'll introduce how these strengths are not only thriving tools but also how they can be used to personalize our wellbeing approach so that it is achievable and sustainable.

These five toolsets have an interlinking and reinforcing effect. Practicing healthy habits can lead to greater energy for positive and social activities and for applying our character and brain strengths, leading to greater vitality. Moreover, we can leverage our strengths, social supports, and positive activities to support our healthy behaviors.

Learning from Experts and Colleagues

I recently edited a short textbook, *Roots of Positive Change, Optimizing Health Care with Positive Psychology,* which provides practical guidance for health professionals based on the science of positive psychology and health. I was also seeking insights and inspiration. How do colleagues and friends with expertise in these areas apply them in their own lives? Pursuing the answers led me to write this book. Their perspectives, as well as my own experience with the evolving and exciting fields of positive psychology and lifestyle medicine, are woven into the chapters that follow.

A few examples of the amazing people I interviewed for this book include the following colleagues. I had the pleasure of chatting with Margaret Moore, a leader in the health coach community, who founded and is CEO of Wellcoaches and has trained hundreds of coaches. The Wellcoaches approach builds healthy habits that are driven by positive visioning and emotions. I also spoke with Dr. Mark Rowe, a family and lifestyle medicine physician in Ireland, who is well-known for his "prescription for happiness" and has been speaking and sharing his wisdom around the globe. I enjoyed another inspirational and delightful chat with Ryan Niemiec, Education Director at the VIA (Virtues in Action) Institute on Character, the leading organization on promoting scientifically validated character strengths.

I invite you to come along on this journey as we explore what they're doing in their lives to harness the tools for thriving. What advice do they have for us?

Does Thriving Apply to Everyone?

As I share my colleagues' stories, I am aware of an important and reasonable question you may ask—how can these healthy lifestyles and positive activities that work for experts also work for you? Sometimes these wellbeing fields are criticized as being available only to those doing relatively well in life.

What about those struggling in major ways, for example, not being able to meet their basic needs such as food and shelter?

I often get this question during my presentations. I respond by emphasizing that although some activities may not be as immediately relevant or available to everyone, others can be, especially those that take little time or resources. For example, regardless of the situation, it's possible for people to shift their mindset to gratitude and try to see what they do have in their lives. This habit of gratitude is an essential positive psychology skill for many (Emmons and McCullough, 2003). Acts of kindness toward others can also lift us emotionally and physically (Nelson-Coffey et al., 2014), even when we find ourselves in unfortunate circumstances.

Research supports that individuals can gain wellbeing from positive psychology-based activities, regardless of their circumstances. According to leading researchers Ed Diener and Louise Tay, "Our analyses reveal that... people tend to achieve basic and safety needs before other needs. However, fulfilling the various needs has relatively independent effects on subjective wellbeing. For example, a person can gain wellbeing by meeting psychosocial needs regardless of whether his or her basic needs are fully met" (Diener and Tay, 2011).

However, I do need to emphasize the role of culture in positive psychology. Early studies suggest that individuals from Eastern or collectivist cultures may benefit from a different set of positive psychology interventions than those from Western and individualistic cultures. Choosing the right activities for your situation (Layous et al., 2013) and culture (Boehm, Lyubomirsky and Sheldon, 2011) can make a difference. The good news is that from among the wide variety of activities found to be beneficial to wellbeing, you are likely to find one or more that align with your cultural preferences and background (Hendriks et al., 2019). We'll look at a spectrum of options here.

A shift in mindset toward hope, optimism, forgiveness, and using one's personal strengths brings a sense of vitality, regardless of our situations. Even when the outer world seems to be completely crumbling, we have the option to look within for our strengths. Taking a few moments to walk outside in the sunshine, sit under a beautiful tree, observe a beautiful flower, or lift ourselves through breath awareness and mindfulness—these simple and short actions can boost wellbeing and are available to most individuals. Even exchanging an authentic hello with a stranger can result in physiologic changes that are good for our bodies and minds (Sandstrom and Dunn, 2013).

How to Use This Book

I highlight the tools that leverage the best elements of a total wellbeing lifestyle. When you look in the mirror, remember you have these five toolsets to draw upon at all times.

If you find yourself overwhelmed or feel you may be on the brink of a dangerous mental and emotional state, please seek the care of a mental health professional. Come back to this book when your mind is in a prepared state.

Feeling particularly eager to armor up and nudge your personal growth? I encourage you to dive in and consider how you can build these tools as your habits of mind and body. The time may be right because you are already actively pursuing a healthy lifestyle and positive mindsets and seek further inspiration or guidance. The way these tools are packaged here may strengthen what you are already doing.

If you use some of these tools but feel like you could be doing more, this may be an opportunity to supplement your approach and develop a more comprehensive thriving package. Try taking small actions right away to reinforce your learning.

Some of you may be struggling and feel you've not managed to build the mindsets and habits you need. You may be feeling a nudge or an urgency to make a change as you see potential challenges up ahead. Perhaps for the first time, you can look at your unique strengths and seek easy-to-access sources of positive emotions. These positive emotions may jump-start you on the journey to wellbeing and growth.

Dr. Mark Rowe, the family practice physician in Ireland whose powerful story you'll learn, summarized the thriving goal well. "If you want to become wise, you need to be able to take care of yourself so that when new opportunities, positive or negative, manifest, you are ready to learn and grow. You are able to grasp that you've got the mental strength, the curiosity, resolve… and the physical and mental vitality to enable you to do whatever it is you're here to do."

I am grateful to my wonderful colleagues, who have been kind enough to share their stories. By hearing from them, you'll gain a special insider's view about how some of the best science can be applied for lifelong happiness and health. Their stories, wisdom, and advice are offered as a springboard for you to create your own personalized toolkit of thriving. I hope you'll be inspired and invigorated to learn more from the resources section at the end of the book and to apply your learnings throughout the full spectrum of human experience.

CHAPTER 1

HOW DID WE GET HERE?

In every day, there are 1,440 minutes. That means we have 1,440 daily opportunities to make a positive impact.

—LES BROWN

Think back on moments in your life when you felt alive and connected to others and had a sense of meaning. You felt you had the energy to pursue your dreams. Perhaps it was during a vacation when you were physically active, hiking through beautiful terrains, exploring a new town, learning a new hobby, volunteering where you could make a difference, or hanging out with those you love. During these moments, you are instinctively embracing the basic elements of health, wellbeing, and positive psychology.

You can intentionally promote that feeling on a daily basis. The science coming out of the fields of positive psychology and lifestyle medicine points to strategies on how we can best achieve it.

The Evolution of Two Scientific Fields of Wellbeing

A panel of medical experts gathered in 2009 to define the burgeoning new field of lifestyle medicine and the knowledge and skills physicians need to offer high-quality services. I was fortunate to serve on the panel and summarize and publish its recommendations. Before this, the term lifestyle medicine had been used in different ways by groups inside and outside of the health care field in confusing ways.

The panelists agreed that lifestyle medicine is "the evidence-based practice of helping individuals and families adopt and sustain healthy behaviors that affect health and quality of life" (Lianov, 2010). The panel emphasized that this practice includes, but is not limited to, helping patients adopt healthy eating, physical activity, and sleep and avoid risky substance use. It also can prevent diseases *and* is the primary treatment for a variety of chronic conditions, such as heart disease, diabetes, and cancer.

These lifestyle activities form the foundation of wellbeing but were incomplete. As lifestyle medicine developed, a new field of psychology was being ushered in—positive psychology. This new area of psychology is defined as the scientific study of human flourishing or the strengths and virtues that enable individuals, communities, and organizations to thrive (Gable and Haidt, 2005). It represents an additional important component of wellbeing.

While lifestyle medicine practitioners are seeking to impact health and quality of life through healthy lifestyles, positive psychologists are seeking to study and promote health and wellbeing as more than the absence of negative mental and physical conditions (Seligman and Cziksentmihalyi,

2000). Many outstanding researchers have contributed to both fields and accelerated what we know about wellbeing. In recent years, many medical and health practitioners have become board certified by the American Board of Lifestyle Medicine, and likewise, many researchers, psychologists, and health practitioners have been trained in formal programs such as the University of Pennsylvania's Masters in Applied Positive Psychology (MAPP) program.

The two fields have progressed in parallel without a lot of cross-discipline collaboration. Yet the interventions offered by each field can reinforce each other to achieve the outcome of total wellbeing and a continuous state of personal growth.

The Link between Healthy Lifestyles, Positive Emotions, and Wellbeing

The need for greater collaboration and integration of the principles and science of these fields became apparent to me during a keynote address by one of the leading researchers in positive psychology, Barbara Fredrickson, at the 2017 World Congress of the International Positive Psychology Association in Montreal. In her gentle but self-assured manner, she emphasized how health behaviors can be influenced by positive psychological processes. I already knew that positive future visioning could be motivating for patients contemplating making a behavior change. I now also learned that positive emotions drive unconscious motivation for change (Van Cappellen et al., 2018) and offer direct physiologic benefits (Kok et al., 2013).

Our emotions, which at times may not align with our thoughts, are more likely to control our behaviors. The Heath brothers developed a nice analogy of a rider on an elephant, the rider representing our thoughts and the elephant our emotions. If the large, strong elephant is determined to walk off the path, the elephant usually wins (Heath and Heath, 2010). Blending elements of a healthy lifestyle with positive emotions gives us the skillpower and willpower needed for total wellbeing.

Moreover, the bidirectional reinforcing link between positive emotions and healthy behaviors is compelling. Not only do positive emotions nudge healthy behaviors but engaging in healthy behaviors boosts positive emotions. For example, individuals who exercise and eat a diet high in vegetables report greater happiness (Jacka et al., 2017). In fact, every major healthy lifestyle modality—eating a whole food plant-based diet, being physically active, and getting adequate and high-quality sleep—has this reciprocal relationship with positive emotions (Lianov, 2019).

The Role of Positive Health

In order to promote total wellbeing, we need to address all elements of health, which are intricately related: mental, emotional, social, and physical health, as well as positive health. Positive health is promoted by positive activities, emotions, mindsets, and social connections based on the science of positive psychology. The term was coined by Seligman to signify a health attribute that produces a longer, healthier life and lowers disease risk factors over and above what is accomplished by traditional health care (Seligman, 2008). Positive health may represent a core mechanism that prepares you to thrive and grow through adversity.

This perspective is confirmed by one of my heroes in lifestyle medicine, Dean Ornish, founder and director of the Prevention Research Institute and well-known across the globe. I was fortunate to work with Dean Ornish as president of the American College of Lifestyle Medicine (ACLM) while he served on the ACLM Advisory Council. Much of the recognition he has received is due to his pioneering research that demonstrated how heart disease can be reversed through diet, namely a predominantly plant-based diet (Ornish, 1990).

But more importantly, he is my hero because he dared to highlight the crucial role of social connection and love in health long before it was considered the standard of care by health practitioners. Social connection and love were regarded as having a role outside the domain of medicine and health care. He summarized the scientific literature on the topic in *Love and Survival*—a book I have recommended to anyone who would listen (Ornish, 1998).

He is a gentle and disarming soul, despite his fame—being a physician to President Clinton and other celebrities, for example. Over the years, he has continued to advocate for the psychosocial components of health and thriving, such as mindfulness.

In a popular TEDx talk, "The Healing Power of Love and Intimacy," he explains that we already have what we seek within us. "Mindfulness (and meditation practices) help us to stop disturbing what is already there. So we are not doing things to build happiness but quieting everything else to allow our existing inner joy and peace to be noticed. However, our culture promotes the opposite, implying that happiness is outside ourselves, that we have to get things, that is, money, power, beauty, etc., from the outer world to be happy and loveable. Then the outer world has control and stress goes up… Yet if we get these things and feel happy, it doesn't last… as if these things are never enough" (TEDx Talks, 2019).

Indeed, when we look into the metaphorical mirror with authenticity, we see our true selves. There we find the strengths we need and can rely on. Instead of spinning our wheels unproductively, we can recognize our inner wisdom. That wisdom helps us to maintain healthy habits, love and connection, and a sense of meaning. By allowing our natural strengths to guide us, we are much more likely to achieve and sustain a state of thriving.

Dean shared that he had to face himself and muster the courage to find his inner stillness, where he could uncover peace, joy, and love. In this stillness, we see our strengths and capacity for habits that will help us build our best selves from the inside out and prepare for our collective uncertain journey of life.

The Positive Psychology in Health Care Movement

As a leader in lifestyle medicine, I have been especially fascinated by the role of emotional wellbeing and personal strengths in a healthy lifestyle. I felt that not enough attention was given to the mental and emotional elements of health. Also, in its early days, lifestyle medicine had aligned with other medical fields as it emphasized addressing patients' problems instead of bolstering strengths. That's surprising, given that leveraging strengths is essential along the path to successful health behavior changes.

In 2018, I was delighted to have the opportunity to convene the inaugural national Summit on Happiness Science in Health Care sponsored by the ACLM and Dell Medical School. At the summit, health care and positive psychology leaders made recommendations later published in two scholarly articles, highlighting the importance and relevance of positive psychology in health care. Dr. Ed Diener, who, sadly, has since passed away, shared his amazing work that ties positivity with health (Kushlev et al., 2020).

I subsequently served as the editor for the first of its kind handbook sponsored by the ACLM, summarizing the scientific link between positive psychology and health and providing practical tips for medical practitioners. I discovered that even greater focus on this element of health was needed to change the practice of health care. We need a movement to promote it. Hence, I established a nonprofit organization, the Global Positive Health Institute, Inc. (GPHI), which provides education, tools, resources, and inspiration for health professionals to implement positive psychology for themselves and their patients.

While the GPHI focuses on education for health professionals, this book is designed for anyone interested in applying lessons from the science of health and positive psychology. I also hope that this book helps you see health with a fresh viewpoint and that you consider discussing with your medical practitioner this approach to health that can lead to a wellbeing state beyond how health is often defined and addressed in health care. Perhaps your questions will inspire your practitioner to learn more and change their approach from mainly addressing problems to facilitating strength-based solutions.

In medical school, we were taught to ask about a patient's "chief complaint," build progress notes around diagnosing and treating that complaint, and maintain a complete problem list for each patient. Instead, the GPHI is promoting an approach in which the health care system asks about and tracks patients' strengths, which are at the core of their capacity to embrace and adhere to treatment and achieve wellbeing.

You can help yourself by focusing on your strengths and also help the health care system by changing the norms of how we interact with and what we expect from our health practitioners.

The Thriving Toolkit

Increases in poor emotional and mental health were recently accelerated by the pandemic and demand effective approaches in health care and in our daily lives. Positive psychology is an essential toolset, as outlined by leaders in the field in a recent review article (Waters et al., 2021), to help buffer against mental illness, bolster your mental health and build your capacity for mental health in a variety of conditions. I've pulled together the thriving toolkit to make the most of these recommendations, use the best healthy lifestyle science, and personalize it with your natural strengths.

Over time, as you develop these habits, you'll feel joyful, hopeful, and physically energized, ready for anything. You might be wondering why I've chosen the five specific sets of tools in the thriving toolkit. We either already naturally harbor these tools or can develop them with intention. I chose them not only because they lead to powerful outcomes but also because they are available to anyone who can devote some purposeful attention to them.

I refer to all five toolsets as strengths because they are self-empowering and pave the way to thriving from a robust and sound position. The first three include activities of both body and mind. The last two involve using our natural strengths. I briefly listed them in the introduction and provide further descriptions here.

1) Self-care health habits—activities that we participate in to take care of our physical health. Healthy habits are associated not only with physical vitality but also with mental health.

   New studies build on old wisdom and continue to emphasize that eating mostly vegetables and fruits and getting plenty of physical activity and enough sleep can turn our mindsets and bodies around in amazing ways. The ACLM is growing at a rapid pace as more and more health professionals see this approach as the most science-based and effective prevention and treatment strategy. "A realization that behavioral interventions and lifestyle change as an essential therapeutic approach to addressing chronic disease is intensifying among physicians and health professionals around the world" (lifestylemedicine.org).

2) Positive activities—activities to take care of our psychological and emotional health, which reinforce our ability to take care of our bodies and have direct physical benefits.

   Echoing the recommendations of positive psychologists, the American Psychological Association (APA) advises making a habit of uplifting activities, such as creating new celebrations, traditions, and meaningful activities. Dr. Earl Turner, PhD, at Pepperdine University also recommends that we "develop the habit of three good things at the end of the day—asking ourselves and family members to reflect on three good things that happened that day, large or small" (APA, 2020).

3) Social support—our relationships, networks, and positive social interactions that support us.

The APA also emphasizes that we find meaningful opportunities to connect with family, our culture, and our community for our wellbeing. The science behind this toolset is based on robust cohort studies—which follow individuals over the long term—that are designed to help researchers tease out what really works. In fact, the ACLM recommends social connection as an important part of treatment and prevention (lifestylemedicine.org). We'll walk through some of the most salient studies (APA, 2020).

4) Character strengths—activities and mindsets that leverage our natural strengths, making it easier to achieve our goals and boost our self-confidence.

Using our strengths to make this a better world can bring us a sense of meaning and increase our wellbeing, as described and promoted by the VIA (Virtues in Action) Institute on Character. This institute states, "Research shows that understanding and applying your strengths can help boost confidence, increase happiness, strengthen relationships, manage problems, reduce stress, accomplish goals, build meaning and purpose, and improve work performance" (viacharacter.org).

5) Brain strengths—activities and mental processes that align with our underlying personalities, as defined by the well-known psychiatrist Carl Jung.

Dario Nardi, one of the leading researchers on the neuroscience of personality (Nardi, 2011), uses the results of his electroencephalogram—brain wave studies—to showcase how to become "brain savvy." He notes that we all have "a consistent pattern of activity, a stable and mutually-reinforcing set of interrelated characteristics to which a person is drawn toward" (Nardi, 2011). We can use these preferred mental processes, which I refer to as brain strengths, to target activities that engage our creativity and improve our workflow and learning processes. The mental processes encompass how we naturally take in information, make decisions, organize our world, and get energized. We'll introduce a few key takeaways from that framework, as described in more detail in my book *My Happy Avatar*.

As you can see, this thriving toolkit focuses on enhancing our daily activities and positive mindsets and using our personal strengths. It offers solutions to the question: How can we rely on ourselves to become emotionally resilient, boost a sense of vitality, harbor fruitful, hopeful, optimistic thinking, and flourish in every aspect of our lives?

Key Points

- The thriving toolkit unites the best science from lifestyle medicine and positive psychology.

- A growing movement of health care leaders is advancing changes in health care that leverage the expanding science of and connections between lifestyle medicine and positive psychology.
- Physical health habits and positive emotions have a reciprocal and reinforcing link.
- Positive psychology activities cultivate a state of positive health that may offer great health protections, wellbeing boosts, and even the ability to grow in response to adversity.
- When we intentionally apply our natural strengths—character and personality brain strengths—we promote our self-efficacy to achieve our wellbeing and other goals.
- Character strengths and brain strengths can be used to customize our toolkit so that using its tools is sustainable.

Activity: Assessing My Thriving Toolkit

Take a few moments to consider your approach to wellbeing and thriving and your metaphorical toolkit.

- Which tools do I find in my thriving toolkit now? How else can I support my current wellbeing habits?
- Which tools could I consider adding or enhancing?
- How can I pay attention to and savor positive emotions while practicing specific health habits?
- How can I boost my positive emotions overall so that I can be naturally driven to a healthy lifestyle?
- Which personal strengths (character, brain, or other self-identified strengths) can I leverage to promote my wellbeing?

CHAPTER 2

WHY NOW?

It is worth remembering that the time of greatest gain in terms of wisdom and inner strength is often that of greatest difficulty.

—DAHLI LAMA

My colleagues and I are igniting a movement to advance positive psychology into health care at a time of great need to expand emotional wellbeing support for all individuals. After the pandemic hit, we saw increasing mental health crises and social isolation of individuals around the world. The percent of people who reported stress in 2020 was up 13.6 percent from 3.9 percent in 2018 (McGinty et al., 2020). These figures were no surprise, as we have been thrust into an escalating level of adversity coming at us from diverse sources—health threats, loneliness, political threats, racism, societal unrest, mass shootings, climate change, or simply fatigue from virtual interactions. I dedicate this chapter to sharing the data and studies that confirm our challenging times and nudge you to take action for your wellbeing now. The remainder of the book focuses on inspirational stories and practical tips.

The Pandemic and Our Collective Trauma

I witnessed these threats in the news and listened to friends who were significantly affected by these increasing events. Although I consider myself fortunate to have a life situation in which I work from home and have a lot of control over the kinds and number of projects I take on, I, too, felt a sudden loss of control and found myself staring into the depths of a completely unknown future when the pandemic lockdown occurred.

We had been following the trends of the early cases in China and then Europe, with an unrealistic hope that somehow the pandemic would not reach us here in the US. We had just returned from a long weekend vacation in Mexico for my daughter's winter break. I'd held a special celebration for my big birthday with a DJ, dancing, and a delicious buffet. Indeed, life was good. We were careful to emphasize handwashing, but physical distancing and face masks had not yet hit our horizon. Our taxi driver shared that he'd heard about one case in a town nearby and was clearly scared and thinking of quitting his work for a while. My partner and I thought that was a bit pessimistic.

A couple of weeks later, my daughter had just settled back into her school routine. I was enjoying a late lunch with a close friend when I received a call from the school that the entire district was closing until further notice. Time froze for me in that moment. Something so basic that I had taken for granted, like my daughter going to school, was wiped out at a moment's notice.

I recall having difficulty grasping what that would mean or visualizing what could happen next. If the schools were closing, things were serious. I had public health training and had learned about pandemics and preventive measures, yet I was a bit stunned. I could not visualize a new daily life. I was so used to planning my life and having a pretty good idea of what would happen next. That guardrail was gone.

As the pandemic rolled out across the globe, billions of people collectively and suddenly experienced upheaval in their lives and the loss of a "normal" future, and millions dealt firsthand with severe illness and the loss of their loved ones. When our level of control and certainty was taken away in an undeniable way... that was trauma. Collectively, we've all experienced mini or major traumas during the pandemic.

When I regained some level of composure, I quickly sensed that I needed to harness everything I knew about health, happiness, and using our strengths to thrive in this uncharted wilderness of life. The early weeks at home with my daughter were fun in many ways. She was asked to read every day until the school could come up with a new teaching plan. She and I had time to paint together. I found myself, with her help, creating a painting of the two of us from behind, arm in arm, as she and I stared into a far horizon—a kind of abyss. There was nothing to paint in the horizon nor the foreground because nothing felt real or stable, but fortunately, we had each other. I also swung into gear to make the most of my training and professional passions for myself and others, including convening virtual support groups.

Stress in America

Many were not so fortunate. The American Psychological Association (APA) warned that we were facing a national mental health crisis with disruptions of work, education, health care, the economy, relationships, and nearly everything in our lives due to the pandemic. At the time of the release of the APA's *Stress in America* report in March 2021, Arthur C. Evans Jr, PhD, APA's chief executive officer, emphasized, "We've been concerned throughout this pandemic about the level of prolonged stress, exacerbated by the grief, trauma and isolation that Americans are experiencing. The survey reveals a secondary crisis that is likely to have persistent, serious mental and physical health consequences for years to come" (APA, 2020).

Three in five adults, 60 percent, say the number of issues America is facing is overwhelming them. Nearly one in five, or 19 percent of adults, said that their mental health was worse than the previous year. They're reporting that they have disrupted sleep patterns and are eating more unhealthy foods, with 42 percent reporting they had gained more weight than they had intended (APA, 2020). Also, even though 86 percent reported living in a household with at least one other adult, 63 percent of Gen Z adults agreed with the sentiment that they feel very lonely. Stressful relationships may add to the loneliness. Nearly one in four adults, or 23 percent, report that they could have used a lot more emotional support in the past twelve months, a significant increase compared to 17 percent in the report one year earlier (APA, 2020).

Other sources of stress surround us. Most adults, 59 percent, regardless of race, report that police violence toward minorities was a major source of stress. This percentage is significantly higher than the 36 percent of adults who said the same in 2016. In addition, 44 percent of people of color reported that discrimination was a prominent stressor in their lives (APA, 2020).

The bedrock of human connection suddenly shifted with the pandemic. Such an unsettling experience and the loss of our "normal" lives combined with uncertainty about the future and the constant drumbeat of the stress in the news led to widespread feelings of being traumatized. We needed a way to navigate this world that had turned upside down.

Lack of Healthy Habits and Positive Activities

The APA's 2021 *Stress in America* report shows that the majority, 61 percent, experienced undesired weight changes—gain or loss—since the pandemic started, with 41 percent reporting they gained more weight than they intended. Also, 67 percent reported they had been sleeping more or less than desired, and 23 percent reported drinking more to cope with stress (Kennedy, 2021).

According to a state-by-state survey coordinated by the Centers for Disease Control and Prevention's Behavioral Risk Factor Surveillance System, only 7 percent to 18 percent of state populations consumed one-and-a-half to two cups of fruits, and only 5 percent to 12 percent consumed two to three cups per day, as recommended in the Dietary Guidelines for Americans (Moore et al., 2015), let alone eating a predominantly whole food, plant-based diet—food consumed in the form closest to its harvested state—as recommended by lifestyle medicine experts (Frates, 2019). Such a whole-food, plant-based diet is not only important for preventing and treating diabetes, heart disease, and other lifestyle-related diseases, but it has also been shown to increase happiness (White et al., 2013).

Along with unhealthy diets, other unhealthy behaviors abound. The Bureau of Labor Statistics reports that only 19.3 percent of the US population was engaged in sports and exercises each day in 2019 (Lange, 2021). Yet exercise is effective in treating depression and improving mood (Cooney et al., 2013). Exercise releases endorphins, feel-good chemicals, and helps produce alpha waves that are linked to a state of relaxation. Exercise is also a natural way to increase a sense of reward, motivation, and pleasure (Frates et al., 2019).

Social Media Overuse

In addition to the struggle with these extraordinary stressors in our lives, we may be adding to our stress and poor mental health through increased use of social media. The COVID-19 pandemic accelerated our reliance on virtual connection and social media, as people had to keep a physical distance. According to some studies, high social media use may be associated with a greater risk for vulnerability to stress and developing mood disorders and feelings of social isolation (Lin et al., 2016). Time spent on social media can be a major distraction from real-life activities that lead to positive emotions and physical vitality.

Moreover, negative interactions on social media can put us at risk. One review of multiple studies concluded that, on the whole, online interactions were associated with both depression and anxiety. They theorized that it was probably because these kinds of social interactions were not high quality. Negative interactions and social comparisons relate to increased depression and anxiety, whereas social support, positive interactions, and connectedness related to lower levels of depression and anxiety (Seabrook, Kern, and Rickard, 2016). Additionally, the more time spent on social media, and the more actively one engages in it, the greater the risk of addiction with potential negative emotional consequences (Karim et al., 2020).

It is also possible that individuals who use social media frequently are less physically active and sedentary, which could add to poor mental health. The blue screens of smartphones used before bedtime can also interfere with sleep (Harvard Health Letter, 2020). Multitasking on several social media apps or platforms while conducting daily activities, schoolwork, and jobs takes our full attention outwards and interferes with peaceful and mindful positive self-reflection. We need more research on this connection between social media use, our moods, and wellbeing. Therefore, we should be cautious and self-aware of our social media use and its potential negative impact. Increasing activities in the thriving toolkit will not only add to our wellbeing but lower our need for spending a lot of time on social media.

Explosion of Isolation and Loneliness

In a national survey conducted by Cigna, the percent of adults who reported feeling lonely increased from 47 percent in 2018 to 61 percent in 2019, reaching an all-time high, and that was before the pandemic. The well-known researcher on social isolation and health, a professor of psychology and neuroscience at Brigham Young University, Julianne

Holt-Lunstad, emphasizes there's robust evidence that social isolation and loneliness are associated with increased morbidity and dysregulation of various biomarkers of health, such as inflammation, and significantly increased risk for premature mortality (Holt-Lunstad, 2020). To put it another way, lack of social connection heightens health risks as much as smoking fifteen cigarettes a day or having an alcohol use disorder. Dr. Lunstad also found that loneliness and social isolation are twice as harmful to physical and mental health as obesity (Holt-Lunstad, 2020). There is ample evidence that social connection reduces this risk (Novatoney, 2019). As we'll see, the social support toolset encourages deep connections and social activities that give you a sense of belonging and has mental and physical benefits (Martino, Pegg, and Frates, 2017). The key is authentic interactions. Even authentic brief hellos with strangers (Sandstrom and Dunn, 2014) in person can be more health-promoting than social media posts by triggering beneficial physiologic effects through what positive psychology research refers to as positivity resonance—sharing positive emotions with others (Major, 2018).

Risky Substance Use

An additional reason that now is the time to focus on the thriving toolkit is the increasing level of substance use. According to the Centers for Disease Control and Prevention, 13 percent of Americans admitted to starting or increasing drug use as a way of coping with stress or emotions related to COVID-19 (Abramson, 2021).

However, substance use is not only related to the pandemic. The National Survey on Drug Use and Health reports that 19.7 million Americans aged twelve and older were battling substance use disorder in 2017, including an alcohol use disorder. That year, 9.5 million Americans suffered from both a mental health disorder and a substance use disorder (SAHMSA, 2019).

Although the data is not out yet, increased rates are anticipated since the start of the pandemic, as emergency rooms see a rise in overdoses. A better way out of stress and into thriving involves positive activities. Positive emotions, engagement, and a sense of purpose and meaning can help people recovering from negative emotional experiences. In fact, positive emotion, engagement and meaning may counter the disorder itself (Butler Center for Research, 2017).

The Veterans' Affairs Whole Health program has had success using an approach that includes healthy lifestyles and positive psychology elements to help veterans struggling with substance use issues, including opioid use (Kenney, 2021). There's also a rich body of work on spirituality and its relationship to recovery and improved drinking outcomes (Krentzman, 2013). These interventions can decrease your risk of turning to substance use.

Increasing Mental Illness

Even before COVID-19, the prevalence of mental illness was skyrocketing, increasing to 19 percent of adults in 2017 and 2018, a rise of 1.5 million since 2016 and 2017. Suicidal ideation among adults increased by 460,000 people from the previous year. The number of people looking for help for anxiety and depression has exploded. From January to September 2020, there was a 93 percent increase over 2019 in the number of people seeking anxiety screening and a 62 percent increase in the number of people looking for depression screening. Many more may have mental health issues but are not seeking treatment. Among people with moderate to severe symptoms of anxiety and depression, 70 percent reported that one of the top three factors contributing to their mental health concerns was loneliness or isolation (Mental Health America, 2021).

The toolsets in the thriving kit, especially healthy habits, such as a predominantly plant-based diet (Mujcic and Oswald, 2016), authentic social interactions (Martino 2017), and activities that promote positive emotions, can have a profound effect as supplements to treatment for those with severe mental illness or as the primary treatment for those with mild to moderate disorders (Waters et al., 2021).

People who are isolated, using substances, or fighting emotional distress are often distracted from paying attention to their bodies and minds. This group can benefit the most from this thriving approach, even by starting with tiny action steps. All of us can enhance our wellbeing by proactively pursuing these activities and mindsets regularly. Even individuals with few resources may be able to find ways to apply a positive mindset and include brief positive activities into their lives.

The mounting levels of stress, dangerous use of social media, risky substance use, mental illness, and isolation and loneliness call for us to take care of ourselves now and prepare for additional tough times.

Key Points

The time is now to build and enhance your thriving toolkit because of increasingly challenging times.

- The COVID-19 pandemic has thrust the world into mini and major traumas; we have collectively experienced this trauma, which may have lasting effects well beyond the pandemic.
- Americans are reporting increasing levels of stress from witnessing negative events in the news, violence, racism, personal illness, and loss of loved ones.
- This increased stress is associated with poor health habits, weight gain, and disrupted sleep, as well as poor emotional and mental health.
- Social media use is on the rise, possibly contributing to depression and anxiety and distracting from healthy habits.
- The percentage of individuals feeling socially isolated and lonely has risen significantly.
- Substance use and mental illness rates have skyrocketed.

Activity: My Emotional Wellbeing

Consider how your recent experiences have influenced your behaviors and current state of wellbeing.

- What experiences do I find challenging?
- What are my feelings, thoughts, and behaviors during these experiences?

- How have the challenging experiences changed my well-being routine?
- What area in my life needs improvement? What support do I need?
- In what ways have I grown as a result of the challenging experiences?
- How can I apply this growth through future difficulties?

CHAPTER 3

STRENGTHS WE CREATE

Happiness lies first of all in health.

—GEORGE WILLIAM CURTIS

Despite the impact of the pandemic and the daily stresses we all experience, thriving remains possible. What are you doing to support yourself, and what else can you be doing to enhance your approach? Let's dive in and take a closer look at the science behind the five strength toolsets of the thriving toolkit. We'll tackle the first three in this chapter. These tools come in the form of tiny and big habits of body and mind we practice daily. We'll introduce the last two toolsets, the internal strengths of character and brain strengths, in the next chapter.

Key Healthy Habits

Many of you may likely be familiar with the wisdom of self-care and what one needs to do to stay healthy: eat a diet high in fruits and vegetables, be physically active, get enough sleep, and avoid risky substances. You are also likely all too familiar with the fact that knowing what to do doesn't mean these habits are easy to build and maintain. The good news is that the field of positive psychology is pointing us in a direction that could make it easier and more fun to engage in these activities and keep our bodies healthy.

I've been avidly following the research on what leads to health and happiness for years and have watched as our collective understanding has grown. Both scientific and popular literature on these topics have exploded. Lots of advice can be found everywhere—books, websites, blogs, videos, and social media about what we should do. That onslaught of information can be overwhelming. Even health professionals can't easily keep up with the thousands of new relevant, scientific publications daily. That being said, a few straightforward guidelines, if followed, will serve you well.

One landmark study examined the "actual" causes of death in the United States, meaning the underlying reasons for populations dying from certain common conditions and diseases (McGinnis and Foege, 1993). These causes apply across much of the globe, as the top diseases leading to death are similar, including heart disease, stroke, and chronic obstructive pulmonary disease (WHO, 2020). The study revealed that tobacco and alcohol use, unhealthy diet, and physical inactivity were the actual leading causes of death, accounting for approximately 80 percent of the premature deaths in the United States. Another fascinating study showed that the combination of unhealthy eating, physical activity, smoking, and alcohol was equivalent to being about twelve years older physically than those who had healthy habits in these areas (Li et al., 2018).

Tobacco remains the leading cause of death, with poor diet and inactivity as close seconds (Kamerow, 2020), even throughout the COVID-19 pandemic. In fact, those with underlying medical conditions caused by unhealthy habits are most likely to have a more serious case of COVID-19 and die from it (Degarege et al., 2020).

Additionally, as both common sense and science guide us, sleep is essential. Many studies show an association between poor sleep quality and diabetes, high blood pressure, heart disease, depression, and mortality (Buysse, 2014). I've been fortunate to be intuitively aware of what lack of restful sleep can do to me as far back as my stressful college and medical school years. Even the night before a major exam, I almost always went to bed no later than midnight. My level of alertness, quick thinking, and boosts in memory resulting from getting enough sleep more than made up for any unfinished exam preparations.

In the decades since that landmark paper on actual causes of death, the field of lifestyle medicine, which I've worked to advance and promote nationally and internationally, has grown exponentially. The six pillars of lifestyle medicine—a predominantly plant-based diet, physical activity, sleep, stress management, avoiding tobacco, risky drug and alcohol use, and social connections—are recommended for preventing and treating chronic diseases, such as heart disease, diabetes, and cancer, now referred to as lifestyle-related diseases (Frates et al., 2019). As you'll see in the next chapter,

I make the case to expand the sixth pillar to include positive activities more broadly.

These habits are not only essential for your physical health but also your mental and emotional health (Blanchflower, Oswald and Stewart-Brown, 2013). A large study surveying eighty thousand British adults showed an association between happiness, mental health, and fruit and vegetable consumption. Studies also show that individuals randomized to exercise for depression versus taking anti-depressant medication get as good or better relief. Physical activity not only improves depression (Cooney et al., 2013) but also increases happiness in general populations (Richards et al., 2015).

Later, we'll hear from Margaret Moore, the Wellcoaches CEO, who shares how she makes self-care her greatest priority. Through preparing and eating healthy meals for herself and her family during one of the most traumatic times of her life when her mother was terminally ill, Margaret was able to persevere, bounce back, and thrive.

Making and Sustaining Self-Care Habits

One scientifically proven strategy for promoting healthy behavior change is associating desired activities with positive emotions. We are more likely to engage in activities that make us feel good again and again. One experience you might have had yourself is enjoying a walk through the woods in peaceful, beautiful, and refreshing surroundings. You also may feel more invigorated after such a walk. When you reflect on this activity later, you're likely to want to take another walk in that environment. Moreover, physical health habits and positive emotions have a reciprocal link and reinforce each other. For example, as noted earlier, eating a diet high in fruits and vegetables is associated with greater happiness levels (Mujcic and Oswald, 2016). The reverse is also true; people who are already happy tend to choose healthier foods (Gardner et al., 2013).

Of course, change only happens when you are ready, and often it is gradual as we experience more and more nudges around us or have an internal awakening. Over the years of reading the science and attending conferences with the world's leading lifestyle medicine experts, I shifted my personal practices to emphasize these habits. Several years ago, I gave a presentation at the Plantrician Project in Anaheim, California, a program teaching health professionals the science of plant-based diet and health, and I stayed for the full four-day conference.

The conference organizers arranged for the hotel to provide all three meals every day with nothing but whole plant-based food. Not only was it phenomenally beautiful with the full rainbow of colors in the salads, vegetables, and fruits, with amazing aromas, but it was absolutely delicious. Being a dessert fanatic, I especially relished the creamy cashew-based desserts and mouth-watering smoothies.

Although I had already been eating a predominantly plant-based diet, that positive experience was the final nudge. How could I ever want to eat anything else? My taste buds were rejecting salty, sweet, and fatty tasting processed foods and fully savoring healthy and delicious flavors. The joyful emotions that sprung up from these flavors energized me to prepare them at home.

The bottom line is that the secret sauce for healthy behavior change is feeling good while doing the behaviors and also feeling good afterward. When we reflect on the positive experiences, we can bring back the positive emotions, which propel us to repeat healthy activities. Moreover, as we have success with our self-care actions, our self-efficacy grows and reinforces the cycle of positive habit change. In chapter 5, I'll share inspirational stories on the power of self-care no matter one's circumstances.

Positive Activities

Activities based on the science of positive psychology represent the second major set of strength tools in our thriving toolkit. What do we mean by positive psychology? It's defined as the study of activities and mindsets that boost positive affect, leading to flourishing. Martin Seligman, who is considered the founder of the field, posited five pillars of positive psychology, including positive emotion, engagement, relationships, meaning, and accomplishment—PERMA (Seligman, 2011).

The P in PERMA stands for positive emotions and encompasses a wide range of emotions, from purely pleasurable ones to meaningful ones. Gratitude practice, such as counting blessings instead of burdens, has been well studied and can lead to a sense of heightened wellbeing (Emmons and McCullough, 2003). Doing acts of kindness, practicing forgiveness, savoring pleasurable experiences, positive reminiscing, and many other activities have been studied as effective positive psychology interventions (Hendriks et al., 2019).

The remaining elements of PERMA are all associated with positive emotions but refer to those elicited by specific activities. The E in PERMA, engagement, also called flow, is a state of mind when you're fully engaged with what you're doing and you lose track of time and surroundings. Making art, gardening, playing a musical instrument, dancing, and other work and hobby projects can lead to this state. When in flow, you find yourself in the sweet spot between being too bored and being too stressed (Chzickszentmihalyi, 1990). Flow involves engaging in activity with a clear set of goals, a balance between the level of challenge it presents and the skills you have to meet that challenge, and immediate feedback so that you know how you're doing.

I personally relish creating art, drawing, and painting. I can spend an entire day getting the shapes and shades just right, mixing paints and various media, layering colors, and more. I often can't think about anything else, as my attention is drawn back to the canvas. Sometimes a dark corner of the painting is too light and needs a dab of cool blue. Other times, a light reflection is not bright enough; a tiny touch of warm yellow can magically make it luminesce. Before I know it, I've missed dinner and it's bedtime.

Engagement at this level is a form of mindfulness. Many people can achieve the benefits of such a state of mind without a formal practice of mindfulness or meditation. We can be fully mindful in our interactions with others. Later, we'll meet Kaylan Baban, a physician who found refuge from the hustle and bustle of the clinic by escaping into an examining room and being fully present during her doctor-patient interactions. She found this emotionally healing for both her patients and herself.

The R in PERMA stands for relationships and social connections. This area of emotional wellbeing and thriving is so important, I've pulled it out as its own set of strength tools that I often refer to as social resources. Our social connections are indeed significant resources that contribute to our lives and wellbeing far beyond what the terms "support" and "connection" relay. The research in the area of positive psychology is most robust, demonstrating how our social lives with family, friends, and even strangers are the single greatest determinant of our health, happiness, and longevity (Vailllant, 2012).

The M in PERMA is for meaning and life purpose. The scientific literature also shows that having a purpose in life has an impact on our sense of wellbeing, health, and longevity. Higher levels of meaning are associated with better physical health (Czekierda et al., 2017). Not surprisingly, individuals with a life purpose and meaning tend to take better care of themselves, as shown through their greater use of preventive health care services and fewer nights spent hospitalized (Kim, Strecher, and Ryff, 2014).

During the COVID-19 pandemic, front-line health workers who were pushed to the brink with the high volume of sick and dying patients coming in have reported that showing up each time for work was fueled by a tremendous sense of meaning. They embraced the meaning of their work in being there to comfort the patients who often had no one else at their side due to isolation mandates (Waters, 2021). When we engage with PERMA in this way, doing good personally and at a community level are in sync.

The A in PERMA stands for achievement. Most individuals strive to set goals for their professional and personal lives and garner a sense of self-mastery and satisfaction when they accomplish them. When we are not successful, goals can be reset to be achievable, to keep us accountable, and help us determine what's important in our lives. Achieving goals that align with our values and feel meaningful are especially motivating and impactful on our wellbeing (Riopel, 2019).

Here, I'm defining positive activities broadly to include not only these key PERMA elements but also other activities and mindsets that improve emotional wellbeing and health, including kindness (Nelson-Coffey et al., 2017), self-compassion (Neff, 2015), time in nature (McMahon, 2015), exposure to sunlight (Lam et al., 2016), activities that lower risk of negative ruminations and loneliness (Layous et al., 2013), and spirituality and religious practices (Chida and Steptoe, 2009). For example, researchers found that healthy people who embrace religiosity or spirituality, measured by their involvement in their religious communities, had decreased mortality rates, even when taking into account other factors (Chida and Steptoe, 2009).

With so many positive activities to choose from, I encourage you to explore them until you find a few that you feel will sustain you. The PERMA framework is an easy way to remember the range of activities. Some you may practice daily or on a regular basis. Others you may try out and set aside for a time when you need extra support. We don't need to use all the tools all the time necessarily. Focus on those needed to achieve a particular outcome. Keep in mind that you'll be more successful in using the tools in times of need when you've familiarized yourself with them ahead of time. Just like during fire drills when we practice our escape routes, being familiar with the tools in advance will serve you well. Not only will ongoing positive activity habits prepare you for those emergencies, but you'll also feel better in everyday life.

We'll further explore several positive activities through the experiences of several friends in Chapter 6. If you'd like to get a jumpstart, check out the websites at the end of the book, especially the Greater Good in Action website (Greater Good in Action, ggia.berkeley.edu), which provides step-by-step guidance for positive activities.

Social Resources

The third strength toolset is social resources. As individuals, we need social connection for our happiness, health, and longevity (Vaillant, 2012). Dean Ornish, a foremost leader in the lifestyle medicine community, has been speaking about the importance of relationships and love for decades. *Love and Survival* was a key early book to highlight studies that exposed the emotional and physical health benefits of relationships (Ornish, 1998). He summarized it well, "The healing power of love and relationships has been documented in an increasing number of well-designed scientific studies involving hundreds of thousands of people around the world." Since then, much more science has confirmed our human need for relationships and social connections for health, happiness, and longevity.

Research points to a clear association between social isolation and greater mortality and illness (House, 2001) through mechanisms such as lower immune system function and cardiovascular disease (D'Acquisto and Hamilton, 2020) and cognitive decline (Barnes et al., 2004). What do we mean by isolation as studied by the scientists? Specifically, we mean living alone, having a small social network, participating in few social activities, feelings of lack of social support, and loneliness. These factors are associated with poor health for all groups, especially the elderly (Tomaka, Thompson, and Palacios, 2006).

On the flip side, research suggests the powerful health effects of social connection. In one study conducted in Alameda County, California, individuals were followed for seventeen years; those who had closest social ties, as well as healthful behaviors, lived the longest (Berkman and Breslow,

1983). One of the most well-known studies of social connection and health is the Harvard Adult Development Study, in which the researchers followed inner-city Boston boys and boys who attended Harvard College over more than eight decades. The researchers checked in with the study participants on a regular basis, asking them about every aspect of their lives—medical conditions, relationships, life satisfaction, and much more. They occasionally brought them in for physical check-ups as well. All that data allowed the researchers to look at a wide variety of factors that may impact wellbeing. Through the analysis, they found that the single most important factor in health, happiness, and longevity is social connection (Vaillant, 2012).

This key aspect of our lives has been noted by wise leaders and celebrities over the millennia. It's a common theme that arises in most interviews as they reflect on life. When Ralph Fiennes was asked about success, he pulled the conversation straight to relationships: "I call people successful not because they have money or their business is doing well, but because, as human beings, they have a fully developed sense of being alive and engaged in a lifetime task of collaboration with other human beings… Success? Don't you know it is all about being able to extend love to people? Not in a big, capital-letter sense but in the everyday, little-by-little, task-by-task, gesture-by-gesture, word-by-word sense" (Whitehouse, 2014).

You might be thinking that relationships indeed impact our happiness, but why is social connection important to our health and longevity? Several mechanisms have emerged in the research. First, our social networks can support healthy behaviors (Umberson, 1987). Our family and friends can motivate us and keep us accountable. Also, social connectivity can boost the immune system. In a well-known study, those who reported close ties and were exposed to the common cold fared better than those who were isolated (Cohen, Doyle and Skoner, 1997).

Another important mechanism is that social connection impacts our hormonal or endocrine system in beneficial ways, such as releasing oxytocin, which decreases the body's stress reaction, including lowering blood pressure and blood sugar (Ozbay, 2007). Most importantly, positive social interactions stimulate our parasympathetic nervous system, the part of our nervous system that is activated when we feel calm and connected with others. This response can be called the "tend and befriend" response when our heart rate and breathing are normal. This reaction has a health protective role compared with the "fight or flight" stress reaction, when heart rate and breathing go up (Kok et al., 2013).

Both the number and quality of relationships are important to wellbeing (Orth-Gomér, Rosengren and Wilhelmsen, 1993). You might ask, what if I don't have very many family members or close friends? Studies have shown that even weak social ties, like talking to the bartender, grocer, or beautician, can promote positive affect and feelings of belonging (Sandstrom and Dunn, 2013).

I hope this peek at the science will motivate you to examine your social connections and relationships and view them as key social resource tools in your thriving toolkit. We'll do a deeper dive into this topic in Chapter 7. Think about what you need to do to foster your relationships. How will you maintain and grow your supports? In what areas of your life are social resources missing? Consider how you can reach out and fill the gaps. Even as you grow your close relationships, remember to interact authentically with people around you throughout the day—it's good for you and them!

These first three strength toolsets—physical self-care, positive psychology-based activities, and social resources—are the foundation for thriving physically, mentally, emotionally, socially, and spiritually. Our physical habits improve our body, brain, and mind. Our positive activities, mindsets, and emotions support our health habits, produce physiologic improvements, and boost our desired happiness—whether that's a state of calm or joyful energy. Humans are naturally driven to do what brings us such positive emotions. In the next chapter, we'll look at the toolsets of our natural strengths that support and personalize our wellbeing actions.

Key Points

We can create, refine, and sustain self-nourishing and thriving tools from three activity-based toolsets:

1) Self-care health habits comprise consistent activities that boost our physical health.
   - Key physical habits include a predominantly plant-based diet, physical activity, adequate and high quality sleep, and avoiding risky substance use.

2) Positive activities promote our psychological and emotional health with direct physiologic benefits, reinforcing our ability to take care of our bodies.
   - PERMA is a framework that helps us remember the five major elements of positive psychology—positive emotions, engagement, relationships, meaning, and accomplishment.

3) Social resources include our relationships, networks, and positive social interactions that support us.
   - Both the quality and the number of social relationships contribute to our wellbeing.
   - Even weak social ties or brief positive interactions with strangers offer health and wellbeing benefits.

Activity: Creating My Wellbeing Strengths

- What are my self-care habits? On a scale of excellent, very good, good, fair, and poor, how would I rate my eating, physical activity, and sleep habits?
- What activities do I regularly engage in to boost my positive feelings?
- What are the relationships that support me in healthy and positive ways? How do I interact with strangers when in public?
- How can I enhance my activities in these areas of my wellbeing?
- What self-care actions would I like to add to my routine, and how will I proceed?

CHAPTER 4

NATURAL STRENGTHS

Nothing can dim the light which shines from within.

—MAYA ANGELOU

The last two strength toolsets in the thriving toolkit go beyond activities that enhance body and mind. They comprise our internal qualities that we can use to thrive. We can rely on these strengths even in times when our outer world feels like it is falling apart.

Each of us carries certain top character strengths, called signature strengths, while adapting and learning to use others when the situation calls for them (Niemiec, 2019). We each also have a preferred way of mentally gathering information and making decisions, based on Carl Jung's work—brain strengths (Nardi, 2011). Brain strengths have another useful feature in that they can also be used to personalize our approach to building healthy habits and positive activities.

Doing so can make the process easier and more comfortable to achieve and sustain.

What Are Character Strengths?

A key element of positive psychology is the use of character strengths and virtues. These are qualities in ourselves that we can leverage in everyday life and during crises. Character strengths, as identified by researchers at the University of Pennsylvania, are referred to as the VIA classification of character strengths and virtues (Niemiec and McGrath, 2019). A well-studied survey is available online at no charge to help identify one's signature strengths—at viacharacter.org. We can develop any of the character strengths, even those that are not our top strengths, by purposefully using them on a regular basis.

The VIA framework includes twenty-four strengths in six domains (Niemiec and McGrath, 2019).

Wisdom Domain

- Creativity—showing ingenuity and seeing things in different ways
- Curiosity—seeking novelty, exploring and being open to experiences
- Judgment and critical thinking—being able to think through all sides of a situation without jumping to conclusions
- Love of learning—being interested in developing new skills and gaining new information and knowledge

- Perspective—having the big picture view and being able to provide wise counsel

Courage Domain

- Bravery—showing valor and not running from threats or challenges and being able to face fears
- Perseverance—being industrious, persistent, and overcoming obstacles until tasks are finished
- Honesty—being true to oneself, authentic with integrity
- Zest—being enthusiastic for life, full of energy, and doing things wholeheartedly

Humanity Domain

- Love—valuing close relations with others and showing warmth toward others
- Kindness—being caring, nurturing, and compassionate
- Social intelligence—having an intelligence around others' motives and feelings and knowing what motivates others

Justice Domain

- Teamwork—being able to contribute to group efforts and being responsible and loyal toward what others expect in a group
- Fairness—sticking to justice principles, valuing equal opportunity for all, and not letting one's biases affect one's decisions

- Leadership—being able to organize groups in order to get things done and give positive guidance

Temperance Domain

- Forgiveness—being accepting of others' shortcomings and giving others a chance
- Humility—being modest and letting one's accomplishments speak for themselves
- Prudence—carefully making choices, being cautious not to take undue risks
- Self-regulation—being self-disciplined, controlling oneself, one's impulses and vices

Transcendence Domain

- Appreciation of beauty and excellence—being able to recognize beauty, admiring excellence in others, and having a sense of awe and wonderment for the beauty in one's surroundings
- Gratitude—being thankful for what's good in one's life and feeling blessed
- Hope—being positive about the future and expecting the best results
- Humor—being playful and lighthearted and bringing smiles to others by showing the lighter side of life
- Spirituality—having a sense of a higher purpose and meaning in the universe and knowing where one fits in the larger scheme

Experts in this science of character strengths promote being aware of one's strengths and consistently applying them. A number of psychologists and coaches highly recommend the use of these strengths, as summarized by Dr. Scott Barry Kaufman, a revered cognitive scientist: "The focus on twenty-four character strengths is highly accessible and of benefit for anyone—young, old, professional, self-employed, unemployed, student, or military—who wants to better understand their potential and learn concrete strategies to bring out the best in themselves and others" (Niemiec and McGrath, 2019).

Using Character Strengths

Routinely and intentionally applying them helps us build habits that feel comfortable and work well in life situations, enhances our self-efficacy, and supports us in achieving personal and professional goals and enhancing our sense of wellbeing. In Chapter 8, we'll learn from an expert in this field of character strengths, Ryan Niemiec, the Director of Education at the VIA Institute on Character, about how he uses them in his personal life.

Besides taking the VIA Survey, we can identify our natural strengths—more broadly defined as any quality that buoys us through life experience. For example, what do others value in you? Ask them what they see as your strengths. Do they often say what a kind person you are or comment about your honesty? When observing others in real life, literary stories, movies, or documentaries, what strengths do they exhibit that resonate with you and feel relatable? When the heroine in a story forgives those who do her harm, do you nod to yourself and agree that's the right way to proceed?

Leveraging our strengths enhances our self-mastery and encourages us to believe in ourselves no matter what. A solid sense of our strengths reminds us about what we can contribute at work and home, day-to-day, and in turbulent times. For example, if you unexpectedly lost your job as a restaurant manager and such work is hard to come by, as occurred during the pandemic lockdowns, you could use your love of learning to develop a new skill and expand your job options.

Being self-aware of our strengths and knowing we can turn to them when maneuvering tough situations gives us the emotional vitality to venture forth into an uncertain world. When your heart hurts from the breakup of a deep love affair, you might be able to apply the strengths of bravery and perseverance to try again for that special someone. Even when the worst-case scenario happens and it feels like the whole world disappoints and challenges you, look in the mirror and remember the virtues you can rely on no matter what.

Identifying Your Brain Strengths

Ever since medical school, when my class took the Myers-Briggs Type Indicator (MBTI) questionnaire to identify the personality type that fits us best, I've been fascinated by this topic. Specifically, I was intrigued with the concept that how we see the world and engage with it can align with certain thought and behavioral patterns shaped by our genetics and upbringing. I have been especially interested in developing a way to use this personality framework to understand our different approaches to health and happiness.

Many of you might be familiar with the MBTI as four letters that represent your personality. This approach seemed too simplistic and somewhat defeatist, implying our personalities are set without opportunity for growth. Moreover, some psychologists are critical of the questionnaire's validity to accurately identify our personalities or explain our behaviors. One criticism is that the MBTI is unreliable because the same person can get different results when taking it at different times (Pittinger, 1993). Others question whether the MBTI can accurately link the results to how they play out in the real world—for example, how well people with a certain personality type will perform in a given job (Gardner and Martink, 1996).

I view the personality framework through a more proactive and growth-promoting lens. Over three decades of studying the MBTI and how experts leverage it, I've learned to appreciate the usefulness not of the personality type categories themselves but, instead, the mental processes that form its underpinnings. These mental processes, identified by Carl Jung (Sharp, 1987) served as the foundation for the sixteen personality types in the MBTI questionnaire developed by Isabella Myers and Elizabeth Briggs (Myers and Myers, 1980). However, individuals may feel stuck with their MBTI results, not seeing room for growth. On the other hand, the underlying mental processes at the heart of Jung's work offer a set of tools that support thriving by allowing us to intentionally leverage and further develop them.

The recommended approach for identifying your Myers-Briggs personality type is to take a proprietary 126-item assessment given by certified practitioners who can discuss the results and interpretation with you. An official online questionnaire is available through The Myers & Briggs Foundation, which can verify the results, and you can make an appointment with a practitioner at the time you sign up. Another option is taking shorter online versions, which are not verified, as long as you keep in mind that the results will be less accurate and use them to launch self-exploration.

If you are mainly curious about your Jungian mental processes, I recommend completing the brief checklist I created, found in the resources section at the end of the book. The checklist gives you a rough approximation of your personality type (Lianov, 2013) and can get you thinking about which personality type might best fit you. Descriptions of the types can be found on The Myers & Briggs Foundation website (myersbriggs.org). Each personality type is associated with certain stronger mental processes—your brain strengths.

Another option is to bypass identifying your Myers-Briggs personality type altogether and go directly to descriptions of the eight mental processes and consider which ones you most often find yourself using naturally. You have lots of experience with your brain strengths, even if you have never been aware of them as part of this framework.

A common analogy compares using your brain strengths to using your right versus left hand to write. A right-handed person can write with the left hand, but with much more effort and a less legible result! Going back to the right-hand feels so much more comfortable and effortless. Likewise, you can become skilled at using all eight mental processes, but many of them will take more energy to apply. On the bright side, this is an opportunity for growth!

Each individual has two out of the eight mental processes that I refer to here as brain strengths, a preferred way to gather information and a preferred way to make decisions. Being aware of them shines a light on them and guides you to proactively apply them to navigate life's challenges. However, under extreme stress, these strengths may not be reliable, and you may need to turn to other toolsets.

The Eight Mental Processes

Information Gathering and Learning

Although we use all four information-gathering processes, which one do you tend to rely on most often? The one you find yourself falling back on the most might be your information-gathering brain strength. Below, I've included two terms for each mental process, first the one in the professional literature followed by the more fun and descriptive term developed by a leader in the field, Dario Nardi (Nardi, 2020).

Introverted Sensing—Cautious Protectors

- Description: linking current information brought in by your senses to detailed memories and reminders from the recent or distant past
- Example: Smelling a delicious apple pie brings back memories of your grandmother and her pies in vivid detail.

Extroverted Sensing—Active Adapters

- Description: fully experiencing physical sensations here and now, focusing on what can be learned from the five senses
- Example: As you walk in the woods, you are fully cognizant of the colors of the leaves, the aromas of the flowers and plants, and the sounds of the birds and your steps.

Introverted Intuition—Keen Foreseers

- Description: trusting your intuition, hunch, or insights
- Example: When considering the safest way to do your exercises in a place you are visiting, you have a sudden insight that you'll be safer at the gym rather than running in the neighborhood.

Extroverted Intuition—Excited Brainstormers

- Description: seeing patterns in the outer world, considering new possibilities or options for the future
- Example: As you stare into the fridge looking at the items available for dinner, you brainstorm possibilities for a creative new dish.

Decision-Making

We need all four decision-making processes, but which one do you tend to rely on most often? That might be your decision-making brain strength.

Introverted Thinking—Skillful Sleuths

- Description: weighing impersonal data and evidence and looking for what makes logical sense
- Example: When deciding whether to support a new public policy to add special designated walking pathways in your neighborhood, you place great value on your

understanding of the logical advantages and disadvantages of walking paths and your analysis of the science behind them.

Extroverted Thinking—Timely Builders

- Description: developing systems that make life easier; organizing the world to address the situation or issue at hand; making choices that rely on outer world organization
- Example: When grocery shopping, you develop a plan for the more efficient route through the store to get all the items you need.

Extroverted Feeling—Friendly Hosts

- Description: noting other people's needs and relationships; considering that impact of decisions on others
- Example: When deciding where to move, you place greater emphasis on being close to your friends and family than practical factors, such as distance from work, the gym, and the store.

Introverted Feeling—Quiet Crusaders

- Description: weighing inner values and impact of decisions on causes and people you consider important
- Example: You buy a hybrid vehicle at a higher price because you strongly believe in doing everything you can to slow climate change.

Using Brain Strengths

As you consider your preferred way of gathering information and making decisions, keep in mind that one of these two is more dominant or stronger than the other. To estimate which one might be your stronger brain strength, you can complete the checklist in the resources section, identify which personality type fits you best, and use that code to look up your "dominant" brain strength in the chart provided.

Another wellbeing tip to keep in mind is that mental processes labeled as extroverted are outwardly focused. Individuals who have an extroverted dominant brain strength are likely energized by interacting with others and engaging with activities in the outer world. People with an introverted dominant brain strength may need more time on their own to get re-energized. Finding the right balance of social interaction can be an essential thriving strategy!

After identifying your brain strengths and spending some time paying attention to your mental processes, you will likely start to see how often you rely on the dominant one. You may see where you could use it more often or balance it with other mental processes. You can also harness your brain strengths to shape your self-care plan in a comfortable and achievable way. My first book, *My Happy Avatar*, and the accompanying individual and coach apps provide specific guidance on how to do that. We'll walk through a brief introduction in Chapter 9.

My MBTI personality type aligns best with ENFP. The dominant brain strength for individuals with this type is extroverted intuition (excited brainstormer). My mind naturally envisions the future. How does what is happening now fit with what I anticipate in the big scheme of things? I learn best when I understand the broader context of why I am learning something. I like to see how some new information fits with patterns of what I've learned before.

In a stressful situation or when faced with a big task or project, I can manage my stress and more easily tackle the project by getting a sense of the overall expectations. If a team lead or teacher unloads a lot of detailed step-by-step information without giving me a solid understanding of the big picture and anticipated outcomes, I get confused and frustrated. On the other hand, someone who has an extroverted sensing brain strength (active adapter) thrives on a project that proceeds with detailed step-by-step instructions and would be frustrated if initially given too much of the big picture without concrete examples.

Carol Dweck is well-known for her work on fixed versus growth mindsets. When someone with a fixed mindset does not do well on a test, they see it as a reflection of who they are without hope for change. When someone with a growth mindset fails a task, they see it as an opportunity to learn and grow (Dweck, 2007). Individuals not well-versed in the MBTI area of psychology are often tempted to use the MBTI to place people into boxes and apply it with a fixed mindset approach, which is quite limiting.

The mental processes underlying the MBTI personality framework can be used with a growth mindset. They can be viewed as tools for taking in information and making decisions to be further developed. This more optimistic, flexible, and useful view allows you to grow your mental processes. As you develop them, however, you'll likely most often rely on your brain strengths, which feel natural and support progress toward your endeavors with less effort.

Being aware of your brain strengths is not only helpful in achieving tasks more easily but is also important in supporting self-compassion when you feel stuck or face a tough situation. Let's look at an example of someone who has the brain strength of extroverted feeling (friendly host) and faces a big decision about whether to help an estranged family member. He may feel less stress when he sees that his natural inclination to offer support aligns with his strengths and values. He can also use his brain strength to discuss the decision in a compassionate manner, especially if he finds he must choose not to offer the requested assistance. When looking back at the situation, he may be more likely to feel good about the decision or how he approached it.

We can use our brain strengths strategically in building our self-confidence, promoting our sense of what we uniquely offer to the world, and navigating tough situations with more ease. Indeed, these strengths, which are often overlooked, are important assets we can rely on when interacting with the world, learning, making decisions, and building habits to secure better outcomes.

Key Points

- Each of us has signature strengths, our top strengths out of twenty-four, that we can use to boost our success and sense of wellbeing and feeling of preparedness for any situation.
- A well-studied online questionnaire can be taken at no cost to identify your signature strengths at viacharacter.org.
- The eight mental processes observed by Carl Jung in his research show up as our preferred ways of gathering information and making decisions. When applied

purposefully, these preferred mental processes, called brain strengths, take less energy and help us achieve our goals more easily.
- Brain strengths can be identified through the formal assessment process by The Myers-Briggs Foundation. They can also be estimated by reading the descriptions and observing which mental processes best fit us.

Activity: My Natural Strengths

- If you are familiar with your character and brain strengths, consider the following:
  - Which character and brain strengths have helped me navigate and thrive through my life experiences?
  - What else would I like to learn about my character and brain strengths?
  - How can I harness my character and brain strengths to grow into my best self and flourish?

- If you are not familiar with your character and brain strengths, you can learn more in Chapters 8 and 9. For this activity, reflect on your strengths, however you define them:
  - What do I consider to be my personal strengths?
  - How have I used my personal strengths for my wellbeing?
  - How else can I make the most of my personal strengths to grow into my best self and flourish?

PART 2

RECOGNIZING OUR STRENGTHS

CHAPTER 5

SELF-CARE STRENGTHS

Physical fitness is the first requisite of happiness.

—JOSEPH PILATES

I entered the profession of medicine not only because I wanted to help people become well after an illness but also because I wanted to help keep them well. My interests later migrated to focus on what keeps people happy as well as healthy. I discovered that physical wellness is a cornerstone for emotional thriving. And I was delighted, as my understanding grew, that my chosen medical fields of preventive medicine and lifestyle medicine represent the foundations of both physical and emotional wellbeing.

Lifestyle as Medicine

Leaders at the American College of Lifestyle Medicine are sounding the alarm that medical practitioners need to discuss with patients how healthy lifestyle habits are foundational to preventing and treating chronic diseases (lifestylemedicine.org). Other health care leaders are echoing this message. Dr. Wayne Jonas emphasized it in an editorial for the American Academy of Family Physicians, in which he clearly expressed how robust studies support self-care therapeutic approaches, like mindfulness, healthy nutrition, and exercise, as the critical steps to achieving wellbeing. "Relying only on the medical system to provide pills and procedures to try to treat these diseases is not enough. We cannot expect to stem the rising tide of chronic illness unless we can design medical practices to promote serious behavior and self-care among patients" (Jonas, 2019).

Indeed, staying healthy to thrive is highly dependent on what we do between doctor visits. Our health practitioners can best serve us by guiding our self-care action plans. Yet many of us can relate to the familiar frustration of knowing what we need to do to take care of our health and not actually being able to follow through. Knowledge and behavior might as well live on different planets. How do we bridge the gap?

Making Habit Changes

One of my heroes in behavioral research is Edward Deci. I was first exposed to his work by reading his book *Why We Do What We Do* (Deci, 1995). I devoured his insights that the core of our behaviors is built on our authentic and autonomous decisions to take action for ourselves. He inspired me with conclusions based on his research. "Human freedom leads to authenticity; it is about being who we truly are. And with freedom comes responsibility because that is part of who we truly are" (Deci, 1998).

He further highlighted that his research confirmed the work of a leading behavioral researcher, Richard Ryan, best known for developing self-determination theory—that people can make changes through innate and universal psychological needs. "All the work that Ryan and I have done indicates that self-motivation, rather than external motivation, is at the heart of creativity, responsibility, healthy behavior, and lasting change" (Deci, 1998).

Over the years, however, I've learned that some individuals have the dedication, personality, and strengths to put their health and wellbeing first, but others are stumped by various barriers. I became determined to look for the most effective approaches to help people overcome barriers to their self-care. Positive psychology uniquely stood out from other approaches as a solution. I discovered how positive emotions can drive our behaviors more powerfully than anything else. That's how I arrived at the doorstep of my current passion for this field.

Let's explore how to propel physical health habits and self-care, the first set of strength tools in the thriving toolkit, through the stories of three colleagues. How did they come to prioritize self-care as an essential strength tool? How do they maintain self-care during everyday challenges, as well as major setbacks and traumas?

A Difficult Balance between Self-Care and Work

In an emotionally moving interview, Dr. Kaylan Baban, Chief Wellness Officer at George Washington University, shared her insights about the need to dedicate oneself to foundational physical habits that grew out of her own traumatic experiences. In the last year of her first medical residency, she had an injury that eventually prevented her from going into a surgical specialty due to her lack of self-care. As a surgical senior medical resident, she was applying for fellowships and making arrangements to go back to work in Iraq, where she had completed her thesis.

"It was very busy, and so there was a period of a few months where I kind of intentionally, consciously said to myself, okay well you know that eating right, exercising, getting sleep and all that you've been trying to maintain throughout residency… that's just not going to happen. You just set that aside." She did not have time to cook at home, so she was getting most of her meals in the hospital, eating what was available, for example, mac and cheese and other unhealthy foods.

She made that choice to set aside her self-care for four or five months, despite knowing she needed to exercise to avoid injury of her unusual joint hypermobility condition. When she was in high school, she had been told her joints were "kind of loose" and that she would do alright if she maintained muscle tone through exercise to keep those joints stabilized. Throughout most of her life, she was active—running, lifting, practicing yoga, and kickboxing.

Unfortunately, after several months of not routinely exercising during that last medical residency year, she experienced a sharp pain in her patella while on a jog. For the next few days, she limped along, hoping it would get better. But when prepping for the operating room one day, she took her shoes off and was horrified to find huge swelling halfway up her leg. She finally had to face the truth, that she had a serious problem and needed to get it checked out. Her patella had subluxed, and she ended up with a severe, chronic pain condition called complex regional pain syndrome.

Her injury required many medical appointments, procedures, and physical therapy. She was trying to keep up with the appointments and her work for a couple of months and realized it wasn't possible to do both at the same time. "I had made it much worse because I'd been continuing to work for a few months, which in retrospect was not super smart. But that was what I did because I thought it was expected of me, *and unfortunately, I believe I was right.*"

This mindset is a common mistake among medical trainees and professionals and many others who continue to plow through heavy workloads, even when experiencing warning signs about their health, wishing the problem would go away! They find it difficult to balance work and self-care, and their workplace may reinforce such an imbalance. Cultures that promote an expectation of long hours can present a major challenge, bigger than an individual can handle when attempting to prioritize self-care. Hopeful signs of changes in health care and other environments are emerging, and momentum is being fueled, in part, by generational changes in what trainees will accept. Advancing the movement to prioritize workplace policies that support wellbeing and self-care represents another essential action step and tool in the thriving kit.

A Turning Point

During Kaylan's last weekend on-call during her residency, she had worked all day Friday dealing with eye lacerations and other major emergencies. As she was putting her key in the door at home that evening, her pager went off. She turned around and went back to the emergency room and was there until Sunday morning. "That was the point at which I started to recognize that this was really a problem... By making that decision and letting myself lose all my muscle tone in my body, eating crap, and not sleeping properly, that created a perfect storm."

She finally had to prioritize taking care of herself, not knowing whether she could finish her training. Once she was diagnosed, she was told that they weren't sure if she would be able to walk again. "That was something difficult to handle. Those were the circumstances where I started to really consciously think about accepting what this is." She made a commitment to do what was crucial for her health, yet she was determined to figure out a way to finish her training. "I was going to keep working on getting myself off of the crutches and focus on one day at a time, which really helps with resilience."

This mindful attention to her health allowed her to pursue as many avenues of self-care as possible that would help her navigate her ups and downs. Physical therapy helped her enormously; she expanded her self-care emphasis beyond exercise to other pillars of a healthy lifestyle like healthy eating. She recalled, "I was a vegetarian from a very young age, and I was attentive to all the aspects of lifestyle medicine." But she had to admit she had let her self-care wisdom slip away. Fortunately, in this recovery period, she was learning to respect self-care as non-negotiable.

Over a period of several years, Kaylan got herself back to a place where she started running again. This was a huge deal because she had been told she might not even walk without assistance again. "I think those [self-care] tools for me have really worked, and I know I've seen them work for others." Healthy habits ultimately helped her recover. And, most importantly, she emphasized the need to maintain these habits. She embraced this area of wellbeing as so absolutely important it led her into the career path of wellbeing.

Although Kaylan's story may be viewed as extreme, the lesson is clear and applicable for all of us. Without maintaining the first and most essential strength tool, taking care of our bodies, we'll potentially sabotage our ability to thrive and achieve our life goals. You may not have a condition that needs such meticulous dedication to self-care and could, in theory, plod along with an unhealthy lifestyle. However, not being as active as you'd like and eating readily available, processed foods, your body will not be functioning at full capacity. Turning your lifestyle around will support you to have a resilient or thriving response to stressful situations that inevitably come our way and assault both body and mind. Seeking life and work environments that promote a culture of wellbeing will support you in this endeavor.

A Mindset to Prioritize Self-Care

Another colleague, Dr. Mark Rowe, a family practitioner in Ireland, about whom we'll learn more later, added further inspiration and encouragement to pursue the goal of taking care of ourselves. He, too, had a demanding job as a physician, which became even more draining during the financial crash in 2010, when he witnessed many patients losing their jobs and their sense of hope.

By 2013, he began feeling overwhelmed by the demands of caring for these struggling patients and not taking good care of himself. "My own emotional bank account at the time was running on kind of empty. And so I learned the importance, since that time, of self-care." While Kaylan's nudge toward self-care was her physical condition, Dr. Rowe's was an emotional one. When hitting this low point, he searched for a solution and was fortunate to find the emotional agility and a peaceful mindset that gives him a sense of inner balance regardless of what was happening in the outer world. Feeling that balance allows one to be keenly mindful of basic lifestyle habits.

"My wellbeing today depends on getting a good night's sleep; I really value my sleep. I leave my phone downstairs." He also believes exercise is among the greatest pillars of health, and he exercises every single day, almost without exception, even if it's sitting on an exercise bike during a patient call. "I would figure out a way to make it happen." He avoids junk food and late-night snacks and tries to eat lots of plants with a variety of colors every day, "eating the rainbow," as suggested by nutrition science (Minich, 2019).

Mark adds one more health habit to his self-care strength tools that we have not yet mentioned. He enjoys the beautiful greenway close to his home and a nearby beautiful world-renowned garden—Mount Congreve Gardens. "I love to get out in nature. A deep connection with nature is really building that sense of inner peace, where there is nothing to stress or worry about and there is nothing to hold on to. It's just a really peaceful place." In fact, research demonstrates the health benefits of spending time in nature for even short amounts of time, including lower blood pressure and blood glucose (Twohih-Bennett and Jones, 2018).

He views this self-care as the starting point for every interaction that matters, including those with his patients. "I can't do the work I do every day to be a caring physician and support people from not a good place myself." He emphasizes that the aforementioned basic self-care elements are nothing magical and anyone can do them. Indeed, these few simple habits or rituals are his "rocks" for health and happiness.

Mark knows that his patients are very interested in what he does and how he acts in his own space. "People are very intuitive and are very emotionally perceptive. They will pick up if you're not taking good care of yourself. It's obvious to others. You're often the last person to see it. You have to align how you are on the inside in your heart and your mind with how you are on the outside."

Self-Care through Challenging Times

A third inspiring and motivating story about prioritizing self-care comes from Margaret Moore. As the CEO of Wellcoaches, a leading organization of health and wellness coaches, she is well-known and respected in the health promotion and lifestyle medicine community. She and I have co-attended and presented at a variety of conferences over the years, where I learned from her that health behavior changes and an emphasis on self-care must be rooted in positive emotions and self-confidence.

In interviewing her for this book, I had the first opportunity to learn how she applies the science of health promotion in her own life. I was eager to explore her experience and wisdom. Not only did I get tips on how she makes a commitment to self-care and sticks with it, but I also found her character strengths, one of the other tools in the toolkit, shining through, including perseverance.

She is currently implementing the same lifestyle habits she has built throughout earlier difficult times. Even when her first husband left her, she never stopped eating well or regularly exercising. She continues to be physically active almost every day and eats healthy food, such as having a snack of carrots at her desk and avoiding takeout meals.

Remarkably, Margaret can stick to her self-care even in tough times. In fact, during one of the most challenging periods in Margaret's life, she discovered self-care as one of the key strength tools in her ability to thrive. When she was in her late thirties, she experienced a family trauma. At that time, her sixty-five-year-old mother had been retired for ten years due to chronic pain and jaw damage resulting from a car accident. Margaret was staying with her parents over a two-month break between jobs, getting ready to move to Vancouver. On her birthday on December 24, she learned that her mother was diagnosed with multiple myeloma.

The cancer was advanced; her mother was greatly depleted and died soon after on Valentine's Day, having spent the last month of her life in the hospital. Margaret feels fortunate that she was living at home, and she could be there for her mom and tend to the family. "I spent all day at the hospital. But every evening, my dad and my brothers were all there. I would make a full dinner. I'm a good cook. After going to the grocery store, I would make something from scratch that took a couple of hours."

This routine kept her going. For many people, having a solid routine they can count on helps them avoid being diverted by major distractions or stressors in their lives. During this challenging time, only two years after her first husband had left her and while her mother was dying, Margaret emphasized her self-care and care for her family. She was proud that they ate a great, healthy meal every night. "I made sure all of us were well fed every night… and we celebrated life. Then I would get up and work out in the morning."

Margaret knew that she needed this routine because she was the primary person advocating for her mother and negotiating with the doctors, for example, to get her mother into a hematology unit, which was not available in her town. Her dad was devastated and did not have confidence around the medical staff to help. "It was magical that I happened to be there at the time she was dying. My strength has always been self-care in crisis… in order to have the ability to do well… and hold my family together."

Positive Habits

I am inspired by the stories and wisdom of these colleagues, who are experts in wellbeing and apply that expertise in their lives. But even for them, finding the right balance of self-care and other responsibilities was not always a smooth road. When life pulled Kaylan away from taking care of herself, she suffered major consequences down the line. Mark ran into an emotional rock-bottom after years of a demanding clinical practice. They had to pivot inwardly to reframe their core priorities. Margaret was fortunate to have built habits from an early age and the natural commitment to use them during major traumatic times.

All three stories showcase how in order to manage the most challenging situations, pursue our passions, and even flourish through tough times, we need to be consistent with healthy habits of body and mind. The good news is that the other tools in the thriving toolkit can support us in doing so. In fact, all the toolsets can reinforce each other, such as positive mindsets and character strengths serving as guardrails to keep us on track with self-care.

In my own life, I have gone through long stretches when my work and responsibilities towered over everything else. Over the years, after long stretches of not engaging fully in taking care of myself, I'd feel an empty sadness and lack of vitality. I find that when I identify elements of my healthy habits that evoke positive experiences, reflections, and memories, I naturally keep them in my daily routine.

I am fortunate to live in an area where I can regularly enjoy the reinforcing sensations of my outdoor walks, the breeze against my face, the refreshing aromas of the plants and trees, and the beautiful array of rainbow colors in the flowers. As we saw earlier, science corroborates the emotional and physical benefits of being in nature (Bratman et al., 2015). I also look forward to delicious meals of savory fresh vegetables, sweet fruits, and spiced grains. And I savor the time I can leave all the hassles of the day behind me and roll into a lovely, dreamy slumber to wake up refreshed, excited about the day before me. These aspects of my day are my safe haven.

My personal experiences and those of my colleagues make the empowering case for the foundational importance of self-care as the first strength tool in the thriving toolkit.

Key Points

- Experts in lifestyle medicine emphasize that our daily healthy habits, such as regular physical activity, a whole-food, plant-based diet, and adequate quality sleep, offer the solution to a vibrant and thriving life. We cannot rely on pills and procedures to be healthy and happy.
- Changing our behaviors relies on our own autonomous drivers and self-care motivators, rather than external "shoulds" and "musts."
- Life can get us—even health care experts—off track from healthy habits, and we need to lean into positive activities to sustain them.
- A thoughtful review and rebalancing of our priorities can help us get back on track and stay on track through authentic action.
- Certain work cultures may not be conducive to fully implementing our self-care; we need to advocate for changes in all work settings that support wellbeing.
- Focusing on the positive experiences and feelings that healthy habits provide can reinforce them in a powerful cycle.
- Self-care through healthy and positive lifestyles forms the foundation of wellbeing and allows us to pursue our passions, persevere through life's storms, and feel a sense of vitality.

Activity: My Self-Care Habits

- What are my self-care habits?

- What situations have derailed my self-care, and how have I gotten back on track?
- What aspects of my self-care can be reinvigorated, expanded, or started?
- How will I use positive experiences and feelings to propel my self-care?
- How will I leverage other tools in my toolkit to support my self-care?

CHAPTER 6

POSITIVE ACTIVITY STRENGTHS

A sad soul can be just as lethal as a germ.

—JOHN STEINBECK

Should activities that bring you joy and positive emotions be part of the health maintenance or treatment plans you develop with your health practitioners? Your initial response might be no. Your doctor and health care team do not have a role in guiding you to achieve flourishing and life satisfaction; their primary role is to treat physical and mental illness, not increase happiness.

Indeed, the latter has traditionally been viewed as outside the domain of medicine. However, upon reflection on the ideas shared here, you might adjust your view. Perhaps health care does have a role beyond managing illness in the form of assisting you with the activities that lead to vibrant health.

The science of positive psychology makes the case that positive activities, the second toolset in the toolkit, have a key role in your wellbeing. This element of health may need a place in our health care, just like managing our blood pressure. And, of course, through our own initiative, we can embrace this element of wellbeing.

Positive Psychology Activities as Part of Medicine

Having been educated in a Western medical school, I believed for many years that, as a medical practitioner, my primary focus was to conduct physical exams, order blood tests, prescribe medications, and do surgical procedures. Engaging in brief, friendly exchanges with patients about what they were going to do on vacation, for example, was a way to connect and help them relax. During psychiatry training, we learned about the medications and psychotherapy that control mental illness. The aim was to help the patient get back to a "normal" or baseline state. Our training did not include interventions to boost happiness, considered to belong outside of the domain of medicine.

Yet I discovered in the ensuing years that if medical practitioners embrace the science of positive psychology and interventions that promote flourishing, they will achieve their primary treatment objectives more easily. Because most chronic diseases stem from poor health behaviors, we need ways to facilitate healthy habits, including leveraging the core driver of behavior change—positive emotions (Kok et al., 2013). Activities based on the science of positive psychology could not only increase health practitioners' success with coaching patients' health behavior changes but with direct physiologic improvements, such as lowering blood pressure, blood glucose, and cholesterol (Kok et al., 2013). I've been advocating for this crucial role of positive psychology in health care for several years. In addition to convening the inaugural Summit on Happiness Science in Health Care and publishing scholarly papers and a professional handbook, I established the Global Positive Health Institute as an educational nonprofit organization to focus on this work. Through this organization and its collaborators and partners, we are disseminating reports of the positive psychology scientific studies, conducting training for medical professionals, and engaging champions to get the word out about the relevance and importance of positive activities for health. We provide practical tips on how practitioners can begin the dialogue with their patients about this topic and tools for "prescribing" positive activities as part of patients' health maintenance and treatment plans.

Key Positive Psychology Activities

The core spectrum of positive activities, called positive psychology interventions in scientific literature, includes activities that promote pleasurable feelings, engage our mind and body, and give us a sense of meaning. Positive relationships and actions that reinforce our sense of making progress toward desired goals round out the list of essential positive activities in the framework of PERMA (positive emotions, engagement, relationships, meaning, and accomplishment) that we reviewed earlier. Additionally, positive psychologists advocate for using our character strengths to achieve our goals and boost our sense of self-efficacy and wellbeing (Niemiec and McGrath, 2019). When defined broadly, as I do here, the field also encompasses other elements of wellbeing, such as mindfulness (Kabat-Zinn, 1982) and time in nature (Twohig-Bennett and Jones, 2018).

Before we walk through a few examples of positive psychology activities, you might be wondering how these kinds of activities work. What are the mechanisms by which positive activities and mindsets lead to health? According to scientific studies, positive affect (that is, a propensity to experience positive emotions) is related to better health behavior, stronger and more frequent social ties, enhanced immune system responses, and changes in hormonal systems that benefit cardiovascular health and lower disease and mortality. Positive affect also indirectly boosts health outcomes by buffering the effect of stress on our neurological and hormonal systems. It even influences our endogenous opioids, our body's chemicals that produce a natural high and lead to healthier immunological and cardiovascular processes (Pressman and Cohen, 2005).

Let's look at several positive activities through the experiences and advice of colleagues in the health professional fields. How do they take advantage of these kinds of activities for their emotional, mental, and physical health?

Mindfulness and Meditation

A colleague who demonstrates a deep understanding of the need to consistently apply these types of activities is Dr. Parneet Pal, Chief Science Officer at Wisdom Labs. She spends her professional time guiding digital and virtual interventions that promote wellbeing comprehensively. She developed her personal habits over many years as her awareness about their importance heightened. At the end of her medical residency, she was grappling with major health issues among her own family members. At that point, she realized the need to take care of her health more completely beyond what she had learned in her clinical training.

"Medical school doesn't necessarily give us that kind of information. So that was my inspiration to dig deeper and to find what I can do that works for me personally, and that I could also bring to my work with clients and patients." She discovered mindfulness, which can be an informal practice of being fully present, and meditation, a more structured process redirecting thoughts to breathing or mantra words. These became powerful wellbeing tools in her life, which grew in importance to her over the years. "A keystone practice that I do is meditation. Every day, it varies. Some days it's five minutes, some days it's half an hour, other days I can invest like an hour or more in it." The greatest benefit she gained was emotional regulation, helping her feel calm and on an even keel during ups and downs.

Other experts in resilience and thriving reinforce the utility of mindfulness. Dr. Robin Ortiz is a physician in internal medicine and pediatrics who focuses her research on resilience. Her most powerful tool for thriving is—you guessed it—mindfulness! "Mindfulness is a trait, more than a state… I don't think it's just an exercise like going to the gym. It's something we can learn, and our brains become adapted to it. Instead of the state of being mindful for twenty minutes a day, it's a trait that becomes inherent in your brain wiring."

She also admits that the results of mindfulness can vary, and only through ongoing practice do we retain an overall benefit. "I've recommended this to my patients... this isn't just like do twenty minutes of mindfulness and you'll feel better. You will, in some cases and in other cases, you'll feel like it was a waste of time. Over time that accumulated practice will put your brain and your state in a place where you automatically pause and have a different perspective. You automatically don't judge, which releases the stress."

Although, in general, many experts in the area of wellbeing find value in mindfulness and meditation, I need to add the caveat that some people do not find it beneficial. In fact, some argue that it can have deleterious effects, such as depersonalization, anxiety, and more (Lustyk et al., 2009). As with all the activities presented here, if you do not already practice it, you may wish to try it. If you find that it doesn't boost your wellbeing, you can move onto the other options offered.

Avoiding Negative Rumination

The next thriving skill is not so much a positive activity, as much as a skill at avoiding a negative one—rumination can spiral us into nonproductive thoughts and a low mood. My colleague, Dani Pere, echoed its importance, offering examples from her life. I worked with her for several years through the American College of Preventive Medicine in Washington, DC, where she served as assistant executive director; we became fast friends. With a fun-loving and kind demeanor, she demonstrates a forthright determination to make the best of all situations by planning well ahead and being prepared. We chatted after she had moved to Boise, Idaho, to serve as the head of the state's behavioral health program.

Dani has naturally adopted the skill of not ruminating about the negative aspects of her experiences. For example, she found this skill useful when her brother, who has many medical risk factors, was diagnosed with COVID-19. "When he told me, I was devastated. That day I was thinking he's going to die. I'm going to have no family. I allowed myself half a day to do it, and then... you're done, no more. It's damaging. You're going to move on. It is what it is. Now you've just got to be there to support him."

Of course, it's not always easy to stop negative rumination, but an awareness to nudge ourselves in that direction can make a difference. Dani and I happened to conduct the interview on the two-year anniversary of her mom's passing from a long illness. She has struggled with guilt and thoughts about what she could have done that might have led to a different outcome. Fortunately, Dani refocused by finding a way to honor her mother." She arranged for a brick to be dedicated to her mom in one of the pathways of the local botanical garden. "A key strength is to not dwell on things. Something terrible happened, you acknowledge it, you absorb it, you think about if there's a way to avoid something similar in the future, but then you let it go." What she describes is an important skill recommended by psychologists for avoiding negative rumination. Reliving in our minds negative events over and over can lead to depression and anxiety (Michl et al., 2013).

Self-Compassion

Positive psychology emphasizes the skill of self-compassion—being kind and gentle with ourselves in difficult situations.

The work of well-known researcher Kristin Neff encapsulates the power of this tool (Neff, Kirkpatrick and Rude, 2007). Someone we encountered earlier, Dr. Kaylan Baban, who shared her story about learning to prioritize self-care in the wake of an injury, also shared how her crisis of imbalance between her wellbeing and her work required self-compassion. She emphasizes how this essential skill needs to be kept close at hand.

"Recognize that, whatever you are dealing with, you may not be able to get through it as quickly as you want. In fact, you might still be dealing with the first arrow when a second arrow comes your way. Your reaction to it can make things even harder." The best practice when life does not go our way might involve giving ourselves permission and mental space to be kind to ourselves. "Self-compassion allows us to come back to the things that we know work for us, our strengths, our tools, and perhaps recommit to those."

Dr. Gia Merlo, psychiatrist and lifestyle medicine physician and friend, echoes the vital role of self-compassion. She has an effortless way of connecting with others, as I witnessed when we jointly led a support huddle virtually for our colleagues at the start of the COVID-19 pandemic. As the huddle participants shared their personal and professional struggles during the initial lockdowns, she gently encouraged them to take it easy on themselves. "We need to show self-compassion and love for ourselves. Instead of focusing on wanting everything to be perfect, just focus on the day to day and what's under our control at any given moment."

She goes on to explain that taking it one small step at a time makes it easier to be self-compassionate. "Focus on this moment and then in another moment focus on that moment. You will have success in this moment, and you will have success the next moment and the following moment. That way on any given day, you can have thousands of successes. That in itself is very empowering, a positive way of approaching the world." Through this process, we can, indeed, discover this thriving strength staring back at us in the mirror.

Gratitude

Another key positive psychology activity and wise habit to develop is to look for the good in our lives even during difficult situations. Researchers have found how a gratitude practice is associated with a heightened sense of wellbeing (Emmons and McCullough, 2003). Dr. Mark Rowe, the family practitioner in Ireland who earlier shared his approach to self-care, emphasized that his favorite positive activity and thriving tool is gratitude. "When you choose to be grateful in the world, more good things come into your world. The more you see things through a lens of abundance and appreciation, the more you realize there are even more good things to see."

It's easy to feel grateful when things are going well and we've had a nice meal and a good conversation. But when life is not going well and we're suffering, we need to turn to an advanced skill of finding gratitude. Mark explains that frequent practice refines this skill. "I've really learned that gratitude is a great habit to cultivate and actively express gratitude for the many things I have in my life. I think it's a great way to see the world, too. It's a great way to reframe, looking back on past difficulties. What can I learn and be grateful for now, even though it wasn't great at the time?" As we shall see later, he harnessed this practice and thrived through a traumatic event in his life.

This potent tool of gratitude can be built through small, simple action steps. "Gratitude practice is writing down three [good] things... Just once or twice a week will do for building it as a habit of keeping a gratitude journal. It takes your mind away from the problems and the negative thoughts and moves you back into your heart and into abundance." Many of his patients who struggle with mental and emotional issues resonate with this advice and find it helpful. "For sustainable wellbeing, a gratitude practice for me is a really powerful idea."

Creative Engagement and Flow Experiences

Although practicing gratitude may be commonly understood as a way to boost our sense of satisfaction and wellbeing, we may not often think about how our daily flow activities can also contribute. Dr. Carrie Barron, a psychiatrist and Director of Creativity for Resilience at Dell Medical School, explains how shifting our attention to engaging in creative activities that facilitate self-expression can help us reframe our internal world and conjure calm, joy, and a sense of meaning. "Whether as spectator or creator, when we are absorbed in music, art, movies, cooking, gardening or whatever, and we feel curious, spontaneous and playful, it's good for our health."

Actively engaging in these activities fits with the E, engagement of flow, in the PERMA framework (Seligman, 2011). Although experts acknowledge that more research is needed on how these experiences can be fully harnessed for health, we can incorporate them into our thriving toolkit now. Health practitioners can even "prescribe" such activities based on a person's values, leanings, and preferences, which may vary widely, such as making pottery or walking a puppy. "Putting it on a prescription pad gives it gravitas and can motivate people to create healthy routines." Some people may find practicing positive activities easier when they view them as a duty rather than an indulgence. However, healthy positive activities can certainly be embraced as a guilt-free indulgence!

Savoring

I had the pleasure of interviewing Ryan Niemiec, Director of Education at the VIA Institute, to learn from his expertise about character strengths, which we'll delve into in Chapter 8. During that chat, he highlighted his wisdom on the art of savoring, another important positive activity tool (Hendriks et al., 2019). In his matter-of-fact and kindly manner, he explained how he often improved his mood by prolonging positive experiences. Indeed, any experience that triggers positive emotions can be extended or even expanded through savoring.

For example, he enjoys eating a bite of chocolate slowly for thirty seconds and really appreciating the richness of the flavor. Even the first sip of chilled water can be immensely enjoyable and uplift his mood. He also makes a point of savoring positive moments with his kids and wife. "My wife and I are sitting out on our patio looking at the trees, and we have an actual moment." He focuses on and savors that moment of togetherness rather than both of them looking at their phones. After that kind of concentrated savoring, the positive feeling can linger long after they have moved onto other tasks.

Meaningful Activities

Ryan recently stepped into the role as a leader of the new Division of Spirituality and Meaning at the International Positive Psychology Association, which he helped establish. It is no surprise that Ryan harnesses a sense of meaning as a key strength tool. The positive psychology literature is growing in the research area of meaning, an element of the PERMA framework, reinforcing its crucial role in health and wellbeing (Steger, 2018).

For example, individuals who report having meaning in their lives may slow the process of cognitive decline in later life and may experience healthy longevity. We can boost our sense of meaning through a variety of approaches. Spirituality and religion have been good sources for many, with beneficial effects on mental health and health behaviors (Koenig, 2012).

Ryan intentionally pays attention to his sources of meaning and life purpose. In addition to the meaning he derives from his family, he finds it in his daily routines. "I've always liked working, and that's how I get a lot of meaning in my life. I connect with people at work, and that's how all the karma comes." The work is both meaningful and creative as he develops new projects, catalyzes new scientific areas, engages in new and different kinds of writing, and makes new collaborations. The art of learning while helping others through work projects reinforces his sense of purpose.

Take a moment every day to consider what activities are meaningful to you and fit with your life purpose. The positive emotions that stem from this kind of reflection and conducting meaningful or eudaimonic activities, rather than simply pleasurable or hedonic activities, are associated with physiologic health benefits (Ryff, 2018).

Being Versatile and Growing Our Skills

These stories from colleagues have brought to light commonly studied and recommended positive activities worth considering in your thriving toolkit. We've seen how they use a wide range of activities—mindfulness, self-compassion, gratitude, savoring, creative engagement, and meaningful activities to thrive. These positive activities are a few examples from an even wider range of activities shown to boost subjective wellbeing—self-reported measure of life satisfaction—and psychological wellbeing (Hendriks et al., 2019).

Having a full spectrum of positive activity tools is handy, as we might find the need for different ones depending on the situation. The PERMA framework is one way to remember some of the key activities, or you might consider organizing the options based on your interests and prior experiences. Ultimately, building our capacity for resilience and thriving depends on keeping all our selected flourishing habits and tools "well-oiled" and ready for action.

My favorites include engaging in creative pursuits, savoring, and conducting meaningful activities. I've mentioned my love of creating a painting or drawing and losing myself in the experience so that all my worries and perceived problems of the world melt away. I extend those positive emotions by reflecting on them when I later look at the piece of art. The most salient example is when I visit a friend of mine for whom I painted a Buddha years ago. I put a lot of my positive energy, my heart and soul into creating that painting, which hangs in her living room over her mantle. As soon as I walk into the room and see it, I get a warm glow and a rush of peace and joy. It's as if my own vital force speaks back to me in the form of that creation.

I can recall that experience any time and relive that same glow. Moreover, the creation of that painting is meaningful in that I made it to support her at a time when her husband was seriously ill and dying. She hung it near his bed, and I'd like to believe she found comfort from this gesture and that he felt the warmth of my caring as the Buddha looked on him during his last days. The three of us embraced the power of our connectedness during this critical time.

When we learn how to use these positive psychology skills well, we can derive a sense of accomplishment and meaning by teaching and sharing them with our children, friends, clients, and patients. The teaching, re-teaching, and connection with others who gain benefits from the thriving tools can deepen and reinforce our own learnings and capacity to flourish.

Key Points

- Activities based on the science of positive psychology can improve our mood and support healthy behavior changes.
- The same activities can lead to direct improvements in our physiology, such as blood pressure, blood glucose, and cholesterol.
- Current research points to an association between conducting these positive activities and improved subjective and psychological wellbeing.

- Practicing mindfulness over time can support the cultivation of a perspective of calm and control when facing challenging or disruptive situations. However, this practice may not be appropriate for some individuals.
- Avoiding negative rumination; practicing self-compassion and gratitude; engaging in creative flow experiences; and savoring and finding meaningful activities are examples of positive activities that can be harnessed on a regular basis for our wellbeing.
- Identifying your own set of positive activities, practicing them, and building them into your daily routines will boost your wellbeing and prepare you for the demands of different life situations.

Activity: My Positive Activities

As you select positive activities, you have a wide range of options to choose from. You might need to nurture a path of experimentation and self-discovery to identify the best ones for you. Some researchers discuss how we need to pay attention to "person-activity fit" rather than randomly engaging in these activities (Layous et al., 2013).

- Which positive activities have I tried or incorporated into my life?
- Which ones have boosted my sense of vitality and positive emotions?
- Which activities will I consider doing more regularly?
- Which new positive activities would I like to try?
- Which ones look interesting? What else would I like to learn about them?

Tips for Building Positive Activities into Your Lifestyle

Activity Feature	Practical Tip	Example
Intent	Purposefully choose activities that fit into your lifestyle	Build flow activities into your weekends
Variety	Vary activities to decrease habituation—lessening of positive feelings by doing the same ones repeatedly	Take a walk in a different park to savor the new aromas and sights of nature
Timing and Frequency	Adjust when and how often you do the activities to optimize the positive effects	To more effectively boost positive feelings, do a gratitude practice every few days rather than daily
Social Support	Identify a buddy to encourage you to engage in positive activities and to do them with you	Ask your buddy to check on your progress
Culture	Select activities that align with your cultural background and preferences	Acts of kindness may be more impactful than gratitude practice for individuals from Eastern cultures
Personality Fit	Choose activities that align with your interests and personality	Take a reflective peaceful solo walk if you tend to be introverted

CHAPTER 7

SOCIAL CONNECTION STRENGTHS

Sometimes being with your best friend is all the therapy you need.

—UNKNOWN

Social supports are essential to our happiness, physical health, and longevity. We all understand this at some level yet can often struggle to make authentic connections and build high-quality relationships. Despite the challenges, developing quality connections is the most vital tool in our thriving kit and well worth our effort and attention.

Concerning Signs in Our Society

Some individuals may not have enough social connections; others may have negative or stressful connections leading to feelings of loneliness and lack of needed support. The 2020 *Stress in America* survey reveals that even though 86 percent of Gen Z adults reported living in a household with at least one other adult, 63 percent of them agree with the sentiment that they feel very lonely (APA, 2020). Almost two out of every three adults, 61 percent, said they could have used more emotional support over the previous twelve months, and almost one in four adults, 23 percent, noted that they could have used a lot more emotional support in the past twelve months, a significant increase compared to 17 percent in 2019 (APA, 2020). Undoubtedly, the changes in our way of life resulting from the COVID-19 pandemic accelerated already-rising levels of stress and loneliness.

These survey results are concerning because scientific studies reveal compelling evidence that low quantity and quality of social ties are linked with a host of conditions, including heart attacks, high blood pressure, slow cancer recovery, slow wound healing, inflammation, and impaired immune function (Martino, Pegg and Frates, 2017).

The Powerful Role of Connection

Research studies have confirmed the human need for social connection and feelings of support to promote our health and wellbeing (Vaillant, 2012). As we saw in Chapter 4, one major, well-done study from Harvard Medical School that followed inner-city Boston boys with Harvard college students over eight decades and looked at a wide variety of factors demonstrates that social connection is the single most important factor associated with our happiness, health, and longevity. These findings have been confirmed by many other studies (Frates et al., 2019).

Experts, including Dean Ornish, one of the most respected physicians in lifestyle medicine, whom I introduced earlier in the book, have been making the case on behalf of love and relationships as essential to health for many years. A few years ago, I had the pleasure of getting a personal tour of Dean's research facility in Sausalito, including his meditation room for groups in the wellbeing program. In his quiet, confident, and disarming manner, he relayed how he lives and what he promotes for patients related to social connection.

He continued to echo this same core message as a keynote speaker at the inaugural Summit on Happiness Science in Health Care that I organized and at the most recent conference of the American College of Lifestyle Medicine. "The deepest roots of healing on a personal and social level [happen] when we can move from loneliness, depression and isolation, which I think is the real pandemic in our culture, to love and connection and community."

Dean emphasized that it is not just whether we have adequate connections but our perception of those connections that matters. We need feelings of authentic connection. "The perception of feeling separate and only separate is the root cause of suffering that ultimately leads to chronic diseases" (Ornish, 2020).

How did he come to this wisdom? In addition to being knowledgeable about the scientific studies that show the link between relationships and health, he personally experienced the impact of not having an adequate social connection. "I am familiar with dark demons because I was suicidally depressed when I was in college. I came as close to doing myself in as one can without actually doing that."

In one of his early books, *Love and Survival*, Dean Ornish bravely shared the details of that stage in his life and how he overcame those inner demons (Ornish, 1998). In January 1972, he was feeling so isolated and depressed that he dropped out of college and went home to recover. At the time, his older sister studied yoga and meditation with Sri Swami Satchidananda, an Indian religious teacher. Upon hearing the swami's wise words during a reception Dean's parents held for the swami, Dean had a great realization that we all carry a sense of peace within us if we just stop disturbing it.

Dean decided to study yoga and meditation with the swami. He had a hard time sitting still at first but eventually caught glimpses of peace and calm through meditation. He went back to college, continuing to practice yoga and meditation, which helped him stay on track. He went on to graduate and enjoyed many great achievements in his early medical and research career. However, he had to admit that he was still feeling some internal turmoil, as he was looking for happiness in the wrong places. "Loneliness... could not be fed by accomplishments and activities." He could no longer believe that if he accomplished more, then he'd be happy. He'd succeeded way beyond his dreams.

He needed intimacy, connection, and love to help heal him. But he had unsatisfying relationships, which he attributes to the fact that both he and the women he dated were afraid of intimacy. He often blamed the women for being unable to be intimate or do what was needed to have successful relationships.

After several unsuccessful relationships, he finally took responsibility instead of blaming them. When things were going wrong, he looked within. After a painful period, he learned to accept and honor himself and others as they were. Only then could he choose to be in a relationship without getting distracted from real intimacy and found true happiness and wellbeing.

Dean's lesson is that we all need authentic close connections, and in our modern society, we must work at developing them for the sake of our happiness and, ultimately, our health and wellbeing. Historically in smaller communities, people grew up surrounded by people in their community who really knew them, saw both their good and bad conduct, and still stood by and cared for them. That kind of social support offers a healing power.

Grow Your Social Support Network

Dean's story is a nudge for each of us to leverage and bolster the social support we have and also seek out and grow the connections we are missing. That means improving communications with our loved ones and reaching outside of our usual circle to expand it.

Different people may feel lonely for different reasons. There's no one size fits all approach to building our social resources. Evaluate your situation. What kind of support do you need? Perhaps you need someone willing to listen without judgment, someone to give advice, someone for a daily check-in, or something else?

Explore how you can use your strengths for connecting and making better bonds with friends, family, and community for a broad set of meaningful social supports. Take action where you think you can fill the gaps, like joining a hobby group or taking a class.

For example, Julene Johnson at the University of California San Francisco was examining how joining a choir can combat feelings of loneliness among the elderly (Johnson et al., 2018). Half of the twelve senior centers were randomly selected for the choir program, which involved a weekly ninety-minute choir session, including informal public performances. The other half did not participate in the choir sessions. After six months, the researchers found significant improvements in two components of the psychosocial evaluation. The choir participants reported feeling less lonely and indicated they had more interest in life, while seniors in the non-choir group saw no change in their loneliness or their interest in life.

While you're building and fully leveraging your social networks, look for high-quality connections in which you and the other person have a mutual positive regard (Dutton and Heaphy, 2003). These kinds of connections positively impact your wellbeing, whether via long friendships or brief encounters. You can purposefully make genuine brief connections throughout the day. One simple action is to give an authentic hello to a stranger you encounter crossing the street or at the store. Surprisingly, these kinds of brief positive interactions are physiologically good for you (Sandstrom and Dunn, 2014). Therefore, even those individuals who have few social connections can derive some of the physical health benefits of relationships.

In fact, the more connections you have throughout the day, the more friendships and the greater the quality of those relationships you have across different aspects of your life, the better. According to researcher Dr. Debra Umberson, both quantity and quality of social connections affect mental health, health behavior, physical health, and mortality risk. Her findings highlight that social relationships impact health through behavioral, psychological, and physiologic pathways. "Adults who are more socially connected are healthier and live longer than their more isolated peers... Social relationships shape health outcomes throughout life and have a cumulative impact on health" (Umberson and Karas-Montez, 2010). A growing body of scientific research corroborates this link.

If you tend to be shy, you might wonder how you can take advantage of these micro-connections throughout the day. Like any endeavor, experiment a little, but also pay attention to your comfort level. Honor your natural self. As noted in chapter 5 on innate qualities, some people whose dominant brain strength is introverted may actually find good social balance and wellbeing benefits from fewer social interactions than those with an extroverted brain strength. Hopefully, future research in this area will uncover insights into these individual nuances in our social needs.

Prioritize High-Quality Connections

If you had to choose, then choose quality over quantity. Make a point of spending time with people who help you experience "positive interpersonal processes," such as sharing laughter, being kind, expressing gratitude, feeling admiration, and being loved (Waters et al., 2020). These experiences are charged with powerful positive emotions that fuel healthy responses in your body and mind (Algoe, 2019). Engaging in discussions in which you share a sentiment or laugh together increases a sense of connection because it helps you to feel similar to your friend (Kurtz and Algoe, 2017). It's crucial to share the good. How they respond when something good happens, for example, their expression of genuine happiness when you achieve a goal, the greater your perception that the person will be there for you during challenging times (Gable and Impett, 2012). When your friends express gratitude toward you, they convey that they are understanding, validating, and caring (Algoe et al., 2019) for you, which is key to high-functioning relationships (Algoe et al. 2019). Hence, science confirms that focusing on the quality of your interactions may be more important than the quantity for your wellbeing.

When I reflect on the high-quality connections in my own life, I realize how much I do rely on them. I tend to be shy in public and do not often find myself exchanging hellos with strangers. But, being cognizant of the vital health effects, I do make an effort. Knowing that I often fall short of those frequent, authentic connections throughout the day, and especially as I spend a lot of time alone working, I rely on my close friendships. I am fortunate to have a number of good friends who live in my hometown of Sacramento, and I am sad that some have moved away. We continue to make an effort to get together and genuinely connect.

I find it interesting that each of my close friendships and the positive interactions we enjoy have evolved in quite different ways. One of my long-time friends—introverted, yet spunky—is quite busy with a large, extended family but always shows she cares by being willing to get together whenever I reach out. While we take a nice long walk, I am comfortable sharing a laundry list of my life events without judgment while she gives caring advice. The way she makes me feel cared for and loved through her attentive listening is magical and healing. In fact, during difficult times, I imagine walking with her, relaying my stories, and feeling better. That positive vision calms me in a deep way.

    My longest friendship goes back to when we were teenagers. No matter how much time goes by between visits, I feel comfortable and cared for when hanging around her. Interestingly, we have not lived in the same town over the decades yet managed to maintain that sense of closeness and mutual caring and validation. She has seen me go through many bumps in the road of life, both personal and professional. When I share an experience, she responds with a depth of truly knowing me.

    She is like a mirror reflecting my life. If I ask her whether I should consider changing jobs, for example, she may recall a time when I faced a similar challenge and how quitting did not necessarily solve my problem. On a recent trip to see her while attending a memorial for one of her family members, I was in wonderment of our mutual caring. While waiting for her at a restaurant, I ordered her meal, and when she arrived, the meal was promptly delivered. I immediately felt a rush of good feelings for being able to care for her body and soul. She ate and we resonated over a discussion about the family we saw at the memorial. I have very few family members and have considered her almost like a sister. Although we may not always agree on a variety of topics, I have a solid sense that we will always be there to take care of each other.

Leverage Virtual Connections Wisely

No doubt, the pandemic has impacted social relationships and caused a greater reliance on phone or video connections.

Besides the obvious lack of touch and hugs, virtual connections present other challenges. It's difficult to make authentic connections when you can't quite see all the nonverbal nuances to understand what the other person is feeling and respond accordingly. When we engage in face-to-face interactions, a lot is conveyed nonverbally through tone of voice, facial expression, posture, and eye contact (Knapp, Hall, and Horgan, 2013). These communication cues may be disrupted online, and we may not be able to accurately convey or receive the positive cues so crucial to building high-quality connections.

Of course, when the situation calls for it, we can make the most of video conferencing, especially for connecting with friends who live far away. Dani Pere, my friend who works in behavioral health at the State of Idaho, explains, "I find it very fatiguing to be on camera. We have about seven hours of [virtual] meetings a day. In a culture where you must have your camera on, you feel a lot of pressure." But when connecting with friends and family, she finds virtual chats incredibly comforting. "We just get together and talk about life… Those types of meetings actually give me energy versus suck energy away from me. We hold meetings with various family members, friend groups and book clubs, and it brings me joy just to see it on the calendar."

In fact, video calls allow us to connect with people all over the globe with whom we may otherwise not have deepened our relationships at all. Many of Dani's relationships have strengthened via her online visits since the pandemic and are increasingly vital. "I have a whole cadre of family members that I talked to once every quarter; we're now talking every week, and… how beautiful. I know so much more about their lives, their children and what's going on in their parts of the country."

Carrie Barron, the psychiatrist and colleague at Dell Medical School whom we met earlier, also leverages the power of her family and friends, both those living in town and out-of-town, by interacting frequently and meaningfully on the phone. "We talk pretty much every day, and that is something that I find very strengthening." She emphasizes her need to talk about deeply personal things, not just touching base or catching up. "For me, the connectivity has to happen on a very deep and real level with a certain amount of authenticity." She is resonating with the advice from the positive psychology researchers of engaging in ways that highlight your common ground.

Conversations with her longtime friends bring back great memories, which they relive together, boosting synchronous positive emotions and health effects, such as lowering blood pressure (Kok et al., 2013). She enjoys "memories like late at night jumping in a pond, or just sitting on the beach and throwing stones in the water on the Long Island Sound. There's something about conjuring those in the memory and sharing them again that's revitalizing."

Use Social Media Sparingly

Before we end our discussion of social support, we need to touch on how using social media fits into the picture. Recent estimates indicate that about half of the global population, around 3.8 billion people, are using these social platforms, and the average user will spend approximately 2.5 hours per day on them (Kemp, 2020).

Some studies suggest that spending a lot of time on social media may be associated with depression and anxiety. How we use social media is also important to consider. If we use it to touch base and arrange to connect in person or post quick updates, that kind of social media use may be important as we build our social networks. However, spending a lot of time venting negative feelings or comparing our lives to others' who seem to have more fun or more friends might be a slippery slope to lowering our wellbeing and ability to thrive (Lin et al., 2016).

One exploratory study of social media's deleterious effects followed a sample of 179 students over one year (Brailovskaia and Margraf, 2017). At baseline, between 0.6 percent and 4.5 percent of participants met the criteria for Facebook addictive disorder (FAD), which involves constantly thinking about Facebook, improved mood after using Facebook, and, over time, a need for increased use of the platform to gain the same mood effects. One year later, 1.7 percent to 8.4 percent met the FAD criteria, with a tripling of individuals displaying "withdrawal" (Brailovskaia and Margraf, 2017).

Several studies show this association between high social media use and depression (Lin et al., 2016) and anxiety (Vannucci et al., 2017). However, the findings are not conclusive. Other studies have shown no relationship between time spent on Facebook and depression (Seabrook, Kern and Rickard, 2016). Perhaps other factors may play a role in predicting anxiety and depression associated with social media use. As we await further studies, suffice it to say that we need to be cautious about our social media use and make a concerted effort to connect offline for quality relationships that help us flourish.

In this chapter, we've emphasized the key role of our social supports and relationships in our thriving toolkit. Throughout the interviews I conducted for this book, the importance of this set of tools was raised again and again. We've learned from savvy health professionals how they create, build, rely on, and savor their social supports to bolster them through thick and thin.

Key Points

- The single most important factor in our wellbeing, hence key toolset in the thriving toolkit, is our social connections.
- We can benefit both from increasing the quantity and improving the quality of our social connections.
- Even brief, positive, authentic exchanges with strangers can have beneficial psychological and physical effects.
- We need to prioritize high-quality connections, especially ones in which we experience synchronous positive emotions that trigger strong physiological benefits.
- Video visits may not be as effective as in-person visits for engaging in positive interactions due to the potential to miss nonverbal cues.
- Scientific literature has suggested that making connections through social media may be useful; however, intensive use of social media may be associated with depression and anxiety.

Activity: Boosting Social Resources

- Which relationships are most valuable to my health and wellbeing because we have frequent positive exchanges?
- What positive feelings do I experience with each of my family relationships and friendships? How would I

describe them to someone else, such as joyful, cozy, warm, and a lightness in life?
- How can I improve my interactions? How can I increase the frequency of positive exchanges in which I feel in sync with another?
- What kinds of support am I missing in my social network?
- How can I grow my social network in areas of my life where I have few connections?
- How do I feel about interactions with strangers and acquaintances? Can I nudge myself to increase genuine brief exchanges?

Exercise:

- Develop a grid of your social network. Along the top, list the kinds of connections you'd ideally like (for example, share an art hobby, take regular walks, discuss work or personal woes, or call in the middle of the night when feeling distressed). Along the side, list the key people in your life.
- Mark the boxes for which you have someone to fill that connection goal.
- Look for the boxes without a checkmark. How can you fill those social goal gaps?

Social Network Grid—Example from someone who lives alone

	Someone to call during a personal crisis	Someone to talk to about work issues	Someone to walk with	Someone to share a gratitude practice
Next door neighbor			✓	
Coworker and friend		✓		
Sister who lives out of town	✓			

CHAPTER 8

CHARACTER STRENGTHS

Go within every day and find the strength so that the world will not blow your candle out.

—KATHERINE DUNHAM

One of the toolsets that we can lean on during challenging times arises from within ourselves in the form of our personal character strengths, as identified by the VIA Survey (viacharacter.org). This questionnaire, developed and tested by a research team at the University of Pennsylvania, helps you identify your greatest character strengths—your signature strengths, out of twenty-four strengths in six domains that we introduced in Chapter 4 (Niemiec and McGrath, 2019). There's no perfect mix of strengths; what's important is applying what we have in pursuit of what matters to us. Moreover, the strengths in the lower ranking are not weaknesses per se but less developed strengths.

The VIA survey is not the only means by which we can learn about our strengths. We can also observe ourselves and ask others for their insights into our broader set of strengths and intelligence. I have learned that applying all my strengths reminds me that even when times are tough and nothing seems to be going right, I can always look within for some bright spots. By leveraging my strengths regularly, not only can I help others, but I can boost my self-esteem and confidence and enhance my emotional health, as well as my sense of wellbeing.

Character Strengths Support Self-Care

Earlier, I introduced Ryan Niemiec, a leader in the field of character strengths, who serves as the Education Director at the VIA Institute on Character. I've been familiar with his work for several years and was fortunate to interview him because I was confident he could provide great insights into the VIA strengths and their impact on wellbeing.

I was excited to learn how he applies these insights in his own life. During the video meeting, from his standing desk in front of a well-organized and massive collection of Pez creatures (fun hobby!), he shared helpful advice and personal examples. I was not surprised to see that he prioritizes and confidently addresses his health using his character strengths. He admitted that although he had always led an active lifestyle, his self-care slowed down after having kids. In terms of health behaviors, "nothing seemed to really stick." Therefore, he created a thirty-day physical activity challenge for himself, including fifteen minutes of cardio exercises every single day. He had told himself, "No matter what, no matter how I'm feeling, I'm going to do it!"

Setting that challenge, committing to it, and having the discipline to stick with it relied on Ryan's strength of self-regulation, which supports self-control and discipline. He also deliberately brought in the strength of kindness, with the goal to be kind and gentle with himself as he built his health habits. He allowed himself to do any type of rigorous activity that raises his heart rate at any time. He self-compassionately accepted the times when the activity doesn't happen in the way he intended every day.

Using his self-regulation strength, he tracked his progress on his smartphone, jotting down on his calendar "cardio" for each day he achieves it. He walked his dog as an additional routine way to break up his sedentary lifestyle of sitting at the computer all day. Harnessing this strength helped him to have self-control and stay on track. "I basically created the [cardio] habit with my character strengths."

He planned to maintain his cardio routine while adding other goals over time, such as meditation practice or eating healthy food. "I'll continue to keep my strengths in mind and use them to be successful with my health, relationships, and other goals. I feel good about my progress. Practically speaking, we could bring specific strengths to any of the pillars of health: diet, exercise, social, and reducing substances."

Indeed, self-regulation can naturally be seen as relevant to achieving and maintaining healthy habits. But how do the other strengths play a role in supporting health and wellbeing? Interestingly, twenty-three of the VIA character strengths (except for humility) are linked with wellbeing (Kaufman, 2015). However, research suggests that certain strengths stand out. For example, in a study of 755 international participants, curiosity and perseverance predicted the strongest increase in goal attainment over time (Sheldon, 2015).

Although these kinds of studies offer promising guidance, Ryan reminded us that further research is needed about how we can leverage specific strengths to achieve our healthy behavior goals. In the meantime, we can look to our signature strengths as potential wellbeing tools. We can purposefully apply them to support our physical and emotional wellbeing. "Signature strengths are one's secret friends and best qualities… We should be more strategic and explore how to expand their role."

Character Strengths Bolster Relationships

Having been successful with his first thirty-day healthy behavior challenge, Ryan not only planned to add other healthy habits over time but also expanded his wellbeing plan to address the most stressful area of his life, his interactions with his wife. He found they sometimes argued and felt tense around each other. He was trying to cut her some slack because she works as a physician and experiences the stress and rigor of seeing many patients. This situation was especially true at the time of my interview with Ryan: during the pandemic.

He decided to make a change and be more kind and gentle with her. Further leveraging his self-regulation strength, he committed to tracking his daily interactions with her on his phone and checking how often he made an effort to be kind and thoughtful. "I was consciously trying not to be negative and not start an argument. If she was showing lots of tension, I would not react or be upset."

In improving his marital relationship, we can see that Ryan also tapped into his signature strength of love. Love, as defined in the VIA character framework, involves the expression of warmth, being a good listener, and valuing connections and can be essential for enhancing any relationship (Niemiec and McGrath 2019).

"I use the signature strength of love deliberately with my kids throughout the day." He works at a standing desk—another health-promoting tool—facing his computer and writing much of the workday. Except for certain meetings, when he locks his office door, his room is open for his family to come during the work day. When one of his kids comes in, he always makes a point to turn toward them and engage fully. His five-year-old daughter will come in, "Daddy, I made this picture for you," and he'll turn, crouch down to her eye-level, and engage with whatever she's interested in. He'll pick up the item, usually a drawing of the family and pets, really look at it, ask her to explain what she has made, hug her, and express gratitude for it.

He believes that even brief encounters like this one, as long as they are genuine, can make a real difference in the bond with his children. "In my stronger moments, I tap into my love strength." He felt reassured that he is becoming a better father and husband when he fully engaged in these brief, but authentic, interactions.

Ryan also shared a story of how he used his strengths during the first date with his now wife. He had been pursuing her for quite a long time in graduate school. Finally, he got her to agree to a date at a nice restaurant. However, she showed up with wet hair and jeans, looking very casual and seeming uninterested. He felt uncomfortable: "Maybe she was not thinking of this meeting in the same special way that I'd been thinking, in fact ruminating, about for six months or longer."

They sat down for dinner, and the conversation lagged. He reached for his strength of curiosity to ask questions, but she was giving one-word answers. He had anticipated that a first meeting to get to know each other over a nice dinner could take hours. In this case, the whole dinner was done in about twenty minutes.

Ryan felt crushed as he observed this meeting that he had been looking forward to for so long fall apart. "We were walking out of this restaurant and my negative spin was going, thinking that this was over and I'd not have another chance." He was battling disappointment, sadness, blaming himself, and asking himself what he had done wrong. His mind spiraled with unproductive thoughts: "This is who I really am. I certainly can't go out with somebody that's really special."

Then relying on his character strengths of hope and perseverance, he pried an opening for a positive approach. "This thought came to my mind literally as we're walking out of the restaurant and I see a little woodchip on the sidewalk. I just kind of kick the woodchip into the bushes, and I say to myself… just give it one more try." With that kernel of hope, he uttered, "Do you want to get coffee or something?" He was totally ready for her to say no, and he'd go home and drink some scotch. Instead, she said "sure" with a happy tone. He couldn't believe it. They met at a coffeehouse nearby, and suddenly the conversation totally opened up. Ryan smiled and posited that perhaps it was the caffeine.

Ryan and his date finally engaged in a deep and wonderful conversation for a couple of hours. By using his strengths, he changed everything. In fact, the rest of his life literally changed because she later became his wife. "The defining moment within that story is the kicking up the woodchip and having that thought to just give it one more try." With hope, you are always looking for the silver lining in any difficult situation, finding the positive. With perseverance, you give hard tasks one more try, and then if you don't succeed, you can let it go.

Beyond Character Strengths

Even as a leading expert in character strengths, Ryan advises us to look beyond this specific framework of strengths to broader definitions of strengths. He encourages us to embrace all our strengths, however we define them. Applying our strengths regularly and in meaningful ways is more important than how we define them. Playing music or sports, spatial and mathematical reasoning, creating art, computer programming, public speaking, and interpersonal relating are just a few examples. These hobbies and work-related skills contribute to our success across many life spheres. Moreover, we can purposefully use our character strengths, like perseverance, to further refine our broader set of skills and aptitudes.

This interview with Ryan reinforced for me the importance of being aware of and using all our strengths personally and professionally during ordinary life challenges, as well as during particularly difficult times. No matter what the outer world throws our way, we can look inward for tools that will see us through and boost our sense of vitality and wellbeing.

Awareness of Our Strengths

Dr. Mark Rowe, the family physician in Ireland whom we met earlier, provides additional sage advice on the powerful effect of actively using one's strengths, based on one's keen awareness of them. He shared how he turned to his strengths during some tricky situations, like when he was making plans for building his clinic. "When I developed the Waterford Health Park back in 2007, I had bought this beautiful thirty-thousand-square-foot convent and we completely renovated and restored it into a primary care facility. Many people have remarked to me in the years since how that took courage." He was self-aware enough at the time that he needed the courage to proceed. Some people thought it was a crazy idea, given that it was such an old building—a legally protected structure—that he'd never get the planning commission required to approve the project. Yet his proposal met with no objections; the whole community supported what he was trying to do.

Through this experience, Mark also reinforced his confidence in his leadership strength and applied it when developing his "prescription for happiness" in Ireland at a time when positive psychology was pretty much unrecognized as a pillar of health. In fact, he sees emotional wellbeing and vitality as a "minority sport" for doctors currently in his part of the world where many have not given it the level of attention he believes it deserves. "But that's okay. I always liked to be a little bit different. So I suppose that made me a maverick leader." Indeed, he built an unusual practice focused on promoting healthy lifestyles, happiness, and living with vitality while emerging as an opinion leader in his medical sphere.

He also values kindness and curiosity in himself and in other people. An essential element of his clinical practice is not high-tech surgery, diagnostics, and treatments. Instead, his own work relies heavily on attentive listening built on curiosity and kind words. "People come to see me, and I try to listen, support them and understand where they are. Listening is really needed in health care now. I see my role in my practice is to support the cultural value of caring. Creating a positive working environment that supports people to be their best selves is so important and, in turn, enables better patient care."

Mark chuckled and added, "That doesn't mean I'm perfect, now, I promise. Far from it, I'm simply a work in progress like everyone else." The takeaway message he emphasizes is the essential need to recognize and apply our strengths. By doing so, we will more effectively harness the opportunities to live the best life we can and become our best selves as we strive to make the world a better place.

In this chapter, we learned from two successful professionals who clearly demonstrate how the third tool in the thriving toolkit, our character and self-identified strengths, can lead to personal and professional flourishing. I was delighted to hear first-hand from Ryan, an expert in the field, how he effectively improved his health and family relationships through the purposeful application of his strengths. It was also enlightening to learn from Mark, who used his strengths to build his medical practice and expand his own self-efficacy, happiness, and wellbeing. The specific strengths they used were less important than the fact that Ryan and Mark intentionally applied them.

Keeping a keen awareness of our strengths and being ready to intentionally use them in our endeavors represents an essential thriving skill. The more we use our strengths, the more we'll achieve our goals, manage negative feelings, promote positive feelings, and boost our overall wellbeing. This process contributes to our preparedness and personal reserves for potential hard times. Like the federal stockpile of emergency supplies, we can turn to our own stockpile of well-sharpened strength tools.

Key Points

- Awareness and active use of our strengths represent an essential element of our thriving toolkit.
- We can identify our signature strengths, our greatest character strengths, by taking a well-studied survey, the VIA survey, online at no cost.
- We can observe ourselves or ask others who know us to identify our strengths of character, our intelligence, and special aptitudes.
- Our profile of strengths is relatively unimportant; what matters is that we actively harness them.
- Making an intentional, concerted effort to apply our strengths on a regular basis can support us in daily endeavors and prepare us for difficult times.
- Knowing that we can rely on our strengths offers the additional benefit of developing a sense of vitality and wellbeing.

Activity: Applying Your Character Strengths

- If you have taken the VIA Survey, what are your five signature strengths—your top character strengths? If you have not, what would your family and friends point out as your best strengths?
- Select one of your strengths and develop a specific plan for how you can apply it to achieve one of your wellbeing goals. For example, if appreciation of beauty is one of your strengths, then taking walks or hikes in a beautiful nature setting may support you to make exercise enjoyable and sustainable.
- Track your progress toward the goal.
- Observe how this strength supports you in achieving this goal.
- Identify another strength that can further reinforce your progress. In the example above, the individual could harness the character strength of self-regulation to ensure she takes her walks regularly.
- Continue this process with additional goals using as many strengths as you can confidently apply.

CHAPTER 9

BRAIN STRENGTHS

———

I was always looking outside myself for strength and confidence, but it comes from within. It is there all the time.

—ANNA FREUD

Of the five toolsets in the thriving toolkit, the utility of brain strengths is the one you likely have least leveraged for your thriving. You may be familiar with the Myers-Briggs personality types (Myers, 1980) but not with the mental processes at the core of this area of psychology (Nardi, 2011) and how to apply them for your wellbeing (Lianov, 2013).

Our brain strengths are the two mental processes out of eight that we most often rely on. According to researchers in the field, each of us carries a dominant one, our main brain strength, and an auxiliary one that complements it (Nardi, 2011). We use one to gather information from the world and the other to make decisions. These brain strengths take the least effort, leaving us more energy for other tasks. Sometimes simply using them can give us a sense of ease and vitality. Moreover, they can also be used to guide our selection of thriving tools and healthy activities and to develop wellbeing action plans that will feel more natural and may be more sustainable.

Understanding the Eight Mental Processes Identified by Carl Jung

In Chapter 4 we introduced the checklist in the resources section that can help you estimate the four-letter personality code that aligns with your brain strengths. Use the chart to look up the dominant and auxiliary brain strengths of that type. If you would like to have a more accurate assessment of your brain strengths, you can sign up to take the Myers-Briggs Type Indicator (The Myers & Briggs Foundation).

Read the descriptions of the mental processes here and observe which ones you rely on the most. Each of us primarily gathers or accesses information either through the five senses—sensing mental process—or through insights and intuition about possibilities in the world—intuition mental process. Each of these mental processes has an external or an internal focus. As before, I refer to the brain strengths with both the term used in the professional literature and the descriptive, and perhaps easier to remember, terms developed by Dario Nardi (Nardi, 2020).

Extroverted Sensing—Active Adapters

The extroverted sensing brain strength focuses on the objective reality, factual and detailed perceptions, and accumulating facts about the external world. Active adapters may seek out experiences that bring out the strongest sensations and may be adept at being fully present in the moment. Examples of activities that use this strength include enjoying physical sensations of exercise and slowing down while eating to enjoy the tastes, aromas, and textures of food. This strength can be highly useful when savoring positive experiences.

Introverted Sensing—Cautious Protectors

The introverted sensing brain strength tends to take in every shade of detail and focus on internal impressions about those details. Cautious protectors may comfortably rely on a wealth of internally stored data from their lives to interpret their experiences. Their perceptions of the world may focus on memories triggered by events. Examples of using this strength include recalling how running outside reminds one of childhood play and being reminded of how the healthy foods one is eating are similar to those served by one's grandmother. Leveraging this strength to conjure up positive emotions may have powerful effects on nudging healthy behaviors.

Extroverted Intuition—Excited Brainstormers

The extroverted intuition brain strength focuses on abstract observations and sees beyond what is in front of us. Excited brainstormers tend to scan the environment for new ideas, possibilities, and patterns, paying less attention to their physical needs than individuals with different brain strengths. Examples include combining exercises learned in a class into a new workout routine and finding an explanation for unhealthy eating patterns during stressful times. This brain strength can incite excitement about the wide variety of positive activities and wellbeing habits one can pursue.

Introverted Intuition—Keen Foreseers

The introverted intuition brain strength focuses on inspirations and insights without a rational explanation or external triggers. Keen foreseers are directed from within by "just knowing" possibilities and anticipated future events. Since they're especially concerned with internal impressions, they may have less awareness of their bodies than others. They may also be drawn to ideas that seem to pop out of nowhere. For example, while thinking about ways to be more physically active, a keen foreseer may get a flash image of jogging on the street where they don't feel safe and realize they need to jog with others or join a gym. Or while thinking of ways to increase their intake of fruits and vegetables, a keen foreseer suddenly gets the sense that the most successful strategy is to eat fruit for desserts. This brain strength supports naturally envisioning how specific positive habits can be incorporated into one's life.

Once we have gathered information about the world around us, we need to decide how to react. Our brain strengths may either focus on the logical or on the value-based aspects of a situation to determine our choice, with an external or an internal focus.

Extroverted Thinking—Timely Builders

The extroverted thinking brain strength draws upon objective decisions, logical principles, and analysis and de-emphasizes personal values. Timely builders may maintain a good sense of the facts and easily restore order to the outer world according to a set of principles, so that organizing, sorting, and applying logical criteria seem naturally easy. Examples of leveraging the extroverted thinking strength include developing a physical activity plan organized around a work schedule; leading a neighborhood walking group, including plotting the route; and identifying science-based criteria for choosing healthy items at the grocery store. This strength can powerfully support restructuring one's life to accommodate wellbeing activities.

Introverted Thinking—Skillful Sleuths

Persons with an introverted thinking brain strength may value objective decisions and emphasize inwardly directed ideas. They may give greater weight to their thoughts and analyses over others' opinions. Skillful sleuths tend to be concerned with clarifying ideas, pursuing practical applications of their analyses, and internally developing logical explanations. With this brain strength, it's easy to decipher, categorize, and figure out how something works. Examples of its application include looking at the pros and cons of different types of physical activity according to prioritized criteria and reviewing the behavioral science literature for the best ways to stay motivated to exercise. This strength can facilitate a deep understanding of the science of wellbeing and its relevance to one's life.

Extroverted Feeling—Friendly Hosts

The extroverted feeling brain strength allows one to more easily make interpersonally based decisions with an emphasis on benefiting others. Friendly hosts may emphasize their values and the impact of their decisions on people over logic. They may seek to create harmonious conditions, readily sacrifice their needs for the sake of others, and strongly support social values. Examples of applying extroverted feeling include arranging an exercise schedule that takes into account a friend's availability in order to work out together or getting input from family members about which healthy grocery items to purchase, making diet changes a family affair. This strength may help one naturally make quality social connections.

Introverted Feeling—Quiet Crusaders

The introverted feeling brain strength makes interpersonally based decisions, filtering most considerations through strong personal values. Quiet crusaders may give priority to their impressions about what's important. They may focus on evaluating the impact of their experiences and actions on highly valued outcomes. Examples of using introverted feeling include becoming more physically active so that one can have the energy to play with one's grandchildren and deciding to ride a bike to work to protect the environment and improve one's health. This strength can powerfully support identifying a sense of meaning and purpose.

These brain strengths can explain some of your patterns of taking in information, interacting with the world, and making decisions. But not all the guidance will be useful. Our mental processes and behaviors are complex and can be influenced by environmental circumstances, moods, stress, and recent experiences. No one theory of our psychological makeup can explain our patterns. Despite these limitations, I have found this framework can provide useful guidance for understanding and modifying our behaviors to help us thrive in relationships, at work and through daily challenges.

Tips for Using Brain Strengths for Wellbeing

If your dominant brain strength is one of the four extroverted mental processes, you likely get energized from and gain feelings of vitality when interacting with others. You likely enjoy social events and take every opportunity to involve others to help you manage stress. If your dominant brain strength is one of the four introverted mental processes, you likely get revitalized when you have time alone to contemplate your internal world and reflections. You may prefer small gatherings with a few close friends (Nardi, 2011).

Another practical thriving tip related to the Myers-Briggs personality types has to do with your level of comfort with planning versus spontaneity—judging (J) versus perceiving (P), which represents another facet of personality. This knowledge can help you avoid unexpected frustrations and stressors. If the checklist and your self-observations indicate that you prefer judging, you may naturally plan and organize your life and the world around you. Such planning is a source of comfort. You may tend to be decisive about what you will do and how you will do it so that you can come to closure and move on to the next task.

On the other hand, if the checklist indicates you prefer perceiving, you may naturally be spontaneous and attracted to staying open-ended about your plans. You may see suggestions, plans, and decisions as preliminary and changeable when additional information comes to light. You may prefer to take in as much information as possible and process all possibilities to avoid what could seem like drawing premature conclusions.

Although brain strengths are shaped by our genetics and environments, we can fine-tune them by applying them regularly and purposefully so we can rely on them when the situation calls for it. This practice builds our self-confidence in a similar way as regularly using character strengths, expanding our options to support our wellbeing, and feeling more ready to tackle whatever challenges come along.

Using Brain Strengths to Guide Selecting Healthy and Positive Activities

In addition to relying on our brain strengths to build our self-efficacy, we can pay attention to them to guide our selection of healthy lifestyle approaches and positive activities. By doing so, we can boost our potential to successfully achieve and maintain our healthy habits.

During a recent interview, Dario Nardi, the leading researcher in Jung's mental processes, whose terminology I use here, shared an example of using brain strengths for shaping his yoga experience. He was curious about exploring this activity through the lens of the different brain strengths. For example, a timely builder may be drawn to yoga because of the tangible, physical sensations and benefits, such as better flexibility. They may also be more driven than others to exercise for the bodily relaxation sensations afterward.

However, they might not be attracted to lengthy visualization exercises that require a lot of internal mental work. They may wonder about the benefits of such visualizations and get more impatient than a keen foreseer. By contrast, a keen foreseer cannot only perceive the benefits of visualization but also enjoy using their imagination to make the experience interesting.

By becoming aware of your brain strengths, you can set goals for an activity that aligns with what feels comfortable and enjoyable to you. Such experiences increase the chances that you will stick with them over time and derive the greatest health benefits. An active adapter may more confidently choose an activity like yoga, aiming to activate and focus on their senses during the activity. They can also "stretch" their mental processes and try some guided visualization exercises while acknowledging that this part of the yoga activity might not be their favorite.

I have found that my dominant brain strength of extroverted intuition, excited brainstorming, supports my well-being activities by allowing me to look for a variety of ways to maintain healthy habits. For example, I am driven to find different opportunities to be physically active, create new healthy recipes, and notice a pattern of connections and successes in my life for which I am grateful. I avoid regular routines that do not provide opportunities for different options, knowing I will quickly drop those activities.

Overuse of Brain Strengths

Although we are focusing on tools we can use over and over to thrive, I need to include a cautionary note about brain strengths. We need to avoid overusing them, which can lead to an imbalance in our lives. Finding the right balance between our brain strengths and the other mental processes, which are not our strengths, is essential to help us achieve certain goals that rely on those mental processes.

Indeed, we can overplay our brain strengths in the wrong context. For example, a great CEO, a timely builder—who focuses on bottom-line efficiency using her extroverted thinking brain strength to easily and effectively direct and organize the people and tasks for the company—might not pay enough attention to others' needs and interpersonal connections. Everyone at work may give her a wide path because she is performing well for the business. However, she may not be gaining the benefits of quality connections! That same person can't go home and continue to use this brain strength in a focused way when interacting with her family; otherwise, those relationships may fall apart.

Excited brainstormers may get so involved in mind activities—writing fun blogs, developing creative videos, or doing online research about favorite topics—that they ignore taking care of their bodies. Active adapters who enjoy the sensations of exercise may push themselves to the point of injury.

Dario warns, "I believe we can all get tunnel vision around our top [brain] strength." He recommends flexing our mental processes purposefully as needed. He explains, "Being right-handed is very convenient for people who are right-handed. They evolved that way, and it's natural for them. But they don't want to tie their left hand behind their back."

In fact, during times of stress, we might be in danger of turning our brain strengths into weaknesses. When we are extremely stressed, we tend to apply our brain strengths in immature and ineffective ways that hinder our wellbeing approach (Quenk, 2002). For example, a timely builder might over-focus on physical pains and sensations during stress. Clearly, this focus leads to greater distress. A friendly host may obsess over making everything perfect for a social gathering, creating stress rather than positivity during the social connections.

Balancing Brain Strengths and Avoiding Stereotypes

Suffice it to say that for the purpose of building and maintaining a complete and balanced thriving toolkit, we need to be aware of our brain strengths and apply them wisely. We can use them regularly to support our wellbeing goals while, over time, balancing them with other mental processes that are not our strengths but are needed to negotiate various life spheres. A timely builder who loves to arrange technical details successfully at work but feels she doesn't have good people skills might need to try out new ways of interacting with people who help her understand their needs better. This process will help her engage in authentic, positive interactions and build social resources

We also need to be cautious about the potential for stereotyping ourselves and others based on knowledge of our brain strengths. Brain strengths are part of our core self—the part that allows us to easily engage in certain activities, like playing a musical instrument or being athletic. However, we should keep in mind the context. That is, we may adapt and behave differently at the office and at home. Also, over time, mental processes that come easily are shaped by our environments.

Due to this environmental influence, the same brain strengths may appear differently in a spectrum of people. Based on leading-edge brain wave studies of hundreds of people, Dario has noted that, at times, individuals with the same brain strength, as identified on their responses to psychological questionnaires, can use mental processes that are not their strengths fairly well. These differences are the consequence of repeated use in their careers. We can adapt and can do an activity well, regardless of whether we find it natural to do. Dario pointed out, "In fact, if they choose a career or an activity that is not naturally aligned with their brain strengths, they're probably bringing a way of thinking about things to their profession that their peers are generally not doing."

As a keen foreseer, Dario's main brain strength is introverted, and he can feel drained by social interactions. However, he feels he is actually pretty good with people. "I'm a different flavor than some other introverts, and that's shaped by my career," a career that has required him to engage with many people through his presentations and teaching of courses. He goes on to explain that the "flavor" of our brain strengths is shaped by culture, society, gender expectations, and the variety of relationships we've experienced over the long term. His interviews and electroencephalograms of people he has studied over decades have highlighted this finding (Nardi, 2011).

Adopting the Spectrum of Mental Processes

It's worthwhile to honor and intentionally use your brain strengths to achieve your goals and support your wellbeing. From that foundation, you can also grow the other mental processes and explore different facets of yourself. By doing so, you can feel vitality and a sense of zest in daily life. Also, life situations may call upon you to be versatile. Being mentally ready to shift as needed is a strength in itself.

Dani Pere, my colleague who moved to Boise right before the pandemic, offered a good example of the advantages of pivoting as necessary. Through self-observation, Dani knows she's a planner, "I am a type-A planner. Coming into December, I would have had the entire year planned, where we're going, what we're doing, what's our financial goal, etc." When the pandemic hit and the future was uncertain, she knew she had to quickly accept short-term planning. "I had to be adaptive... I had to ease into that uncomfortableness of uncertainty and having flexibility of mind." For example, she had to cancel business and vacation trips and stay open to when she could travel again.

To the extent we can leverage our brain strengths toward our personal and professional success, we should. However, leaning on them when the situation calls for other approaches may become a barrier to our success and wellbeing and may cause undue stress. We need to remember that stressful situations might lead us to use our brain strengths in immature or ineffective ways (Quenk, 1993). So when we are extremely stressed, we need to look to other tools in our toolkit.

Brain strengths, whether through formal MBTI assessments or through self-observation, provide another lens for viewing our innate strengths. While being cognizant not to overuse them or rely on them inappropriately, we can wisely apply them as an essential toolset in our thriving toolkit.

Key Points

- Eight mental processes, identified by Carl Jung, encompass gathering information and making decisions.
- We each have a dominant and an auxiliary brain strength shaped by our genetics and early upbringing.
- We can identify our strengths through self-observation, reflection, and tools, such as the Myers-Briggs Type Indicator.
- We can experience success and vitality by intentionally using these brain strengths to achieve our goals.
- Over-reliance on our particular brain strengths can lead to limited and ineffective responses to some of life's demands.
- We can "stretch" our brains by intentionally using mental processes that are not our best strengths, allowing us to be versatile throughout life experiences.

Activity: My Brain Strengths

The resources section at the end of the book provides a checklist and chart to help you identify your information-gathering and decision-making brain strengths.

- What is my information-gathering brain strength?
    - How can I use it to support a self-care activity?
- What is my decision-making brain strength?
    - How can I use it to support a self-care activity?

- Which is my dominant brain strength, and which one is my auxiliary one?
- Is my dominant brain strength extroverted or introverted? How can I use this information in planning my social interactions?
- How can I leverage my brain strengths to boost the other tools in my toolkit?

PART 3

APPLYING OUR STRENGTHS

CHAPTER 10

RELIABLE STRENGTHS DURING TRAUMA

Life is not about waiting for the storms to pass. It's about learning how to dance in the rain.

—VIVIAN GREENE

We all experience traumas, small or large, at some point in our lives. Knowing this can motivate us to continually apply and become well-versed in using the strength tools in our thriving toolkit. Then when a traumatic event comes along, we cannot only weather it but also grow from it.

How do you apply these tools during trauma? Look for what is most relevant at the time. When your entire world seems to be falling apart and you can do nothing to fix your problems, that is the crucial time to turn to your character strengths (Niemiec and McGrath, 2019). Check to see which of your strengths can be leveraged to help repair the situation or shield you against the negative emotions that were triggered. Remind yourself about your good traits and take comfort in that knowledge, paving the way to self-compassion, one of the tools in the positive activity toolset.

Let's explore three stories of how character strengths have supported individuals through traumas, as well as led them to thrive and grow beyond those traumas.

Becoming a Mother by Harnessing Perseverance, Forgiveness, and Bravery

One of the greatest traumas of my life occurred when my mother was not supportive of my adopting a child. In 2011, my husband and I had completed the adoption process and were getting ready to go to China to meet our daughter for the first time. The day before our trip, my mother had a total meltdown and I felt paralyzed, especially because my husband at the time was not fully on board with the adoption. I felt scared and all alone.

This decision to adopt, the biggest of my life, was not supported by two of the most important people in my life, not to mention friends who had also expressed doubts. Without that support, I felt like I could not move forward. At the last minute, on the way to the airport, I called the adoption agency and told them that we had changed our minds. My heart felt like it had been beaten up by everyone around me. I felt lost with nothing to lean on.

My husband wanted to go to China anyway since the tickets were paid for and arrangements for other travel and touring had already been made. Throughout that trip, I barely smiled or spoke. In pictures, I looked pale as a ghost. It's as if I had lost my soul.

I put that whole traumatic incident out of my mind and marched forward with my life. But from deep inside me bubbled up a reminder that two of my signature strengths are forgiveness and perseverance. After a few months, I forgave my mother and my husband, and I started to revisit the idea of adopting.

I also turned to hope, a character strength that I do not often use but find powerful. Despite everything we had been through, I became hopeful that I could convince my husband to try again. This time, we would leave everyone else out of the decision so that they would not weigh us down again. Miraculously, with the help of another agency, I identified a little girl that seemed right for us, and I garnered my husband's support.

Back in China, the adoption process went smoothly. I recall my nervousness the day we were to meet our daughter as I paced in our hotel room, occasionally looking out at a snow-covered pond below and mist in the air. What would motherhood be like? I had no idea but was sure my life would never be the same again.

The strong excitement I felt when I first caught a glimpse of her reverberates with me always. Several families waited to meet their adopted children in the hotel lobby. "There she is!" I squealed as an orphanage caregiver came through the lobby door with three young children. "How do you know?" my husband inquired. We had only seen a picture of her when she was much younger. "I just know!" Indeed, I was right. We embraced her fully, heart and soul, from that moment; even my reticent husband immediately fell in love.

A few days after returning home as a new family of three, I had to face my mother. We had led her to believe we loved China so much that we were going on a second tour to visit additional regions. My mother represented the greatest emotional obstacle, as she always had such a stronghold over me. But I had used my strengths of forgiveness and perseverance successfully thus far, and I knew I could rely on these strengths again. I also had to muster another character strength, bravery, when I brought my daughter to meet my mother for the first time, unannounced.

I remember those first few moments of my mother and daughter meeting in detail and can relive it as if watching a video in slow motion. I walked along the concrete pathway that borders one side of my mother's house, feeling the warm sunshine on my back and the weight of my little girl in my arms, sensing how fast my heart was racing and hearing her little giggle. Most importantly, I felt comfort in my new reality of being a mother myself and fully owning that decision. As nervous as I was, I felt fully grounded.

As I followed the path that curved around to the back of the house where I knew my mother was gardening, I pondered the unknown. How would my stern, judgmental mother react? I was standing at the intersection of my two greatest loves, my mother and my daughter. I needed them to love each other, as I loved them both.

As I reached the back garden, I caught a glimpse of my mother bent over a table of tomatoes. I said, "Mom... Mom, I want you to meet my daughter." As she slowly turned around, I was laser focused on every muscle in her face. What would the expression be? I saw the corner of her mouth slowly curl upward when she surveyed my daughter, and I felt a tingle of relief. I knew everything would be okay. We would all be a real family at last.

I look back at that momentous occasion and recognize the bravery it took to follow my dream, despite so much opposition and judgment. My self-confidence and self-respect continue to grow because I broke the chains that bound me to my mother and truly grew up by taking that big risk, one very worthwhile. My daughter is the love of my life. This dream of becoming a mother became a reality because I leaned into both my signature strengths, as well as other character strengths, to navigate this event.

Love, Kindness, and Gratitude during the Pandemic

Margaret Moore, who earlier shared her experience with the loss of her mother, advises that we take time to feel *all* our emotions during traumatic events. Then we can grow through them. She highlighted the trauma the whole world experienced with the pandemic. Margaret admitted that when Andrea Bocelli sang "Amazing Grace" on Easter in the early months of the pandemic, she wept for the world and also people in her life who were suffering. She had a physician client who was on a ventilator for thirty-five days. "I wept, and then I wrote a blog called 'Leading with Amazing Grace,' based on the lyrics. I felt it deeply, and I poured my heart into this little article, one of the best things I've written." This blog drew upon her character strengths of love, kindness, and social intelligence.

In order to grow, shifting one's mindset to see the meaning in life's trials is essential. Margaret emphasizes growth emerges from trauma when we find forgiveness, gratitude, appreciation of the beauty in small things, savoring deeper connections, and looking for hopeful new possibilities. "I make space to spot those things, emerging like little green shoots… And then, harvesting that; turning the trauma into growth."

Margaret reminds us that we need to refocus our mindsets and harness empowered approaches for tackling any goal or adversity, just as I had to do to achieve my dream of having a family. Intentional use of character strengths, whether these are your signature strengths or not, can support the process she describes. Regular application and a powerful commitment to leverage your strengths can carry you through tough times and build a state of mind ready for anything life brings along.

Hope, Gratitude, Forgiveness, and Creativity to Start Over

One of the most powerful stories I heard in doing research for this book came from Dr. Mark Rowe. We met him earlier when I showcased him as a physician who promotes his Prescription for Happiness to patients and groups around the world with straightforward advice to get enough sleep, get plenty of exercise, lay off the junk food, do things that align with your values, and spend time with happy people. "It's very actionable. It's not rocket science. And it's therefore very usable." By using the character strengths of self-regulation and perseverance, we can follow his wise counsel and prepare the body and mind to thrive through terrible events, like the one he experienced.

Two decades ago, he had set up his medical practice above a shop close to where he had grown up in Waterford. "We put everything, our heart and souls, into the place." He even moved furniture from his own home there. "We were very proud of everything, we worked hard, and everything was going really well."

Early one morning a year later, a guard knocked on Mark's front door and anxiously said, "You better come quickly; your practice is on fire." He got dressed and rushed over there to see the fire brigade had already been there and had done what they could. The neighbors were standing around watching.

"I could see that everything I'd worked so hard for had gone up in smoke in front of my eyes. About an hour later, we went into the premises, and as I walked up the stairs, I'll never forget the smell, this kind of mixture of charred wood, burned rubber, and smoke. I remember seeing what looked like a red party balloon on the wall. But when I got to the top of the stairs, I realized it was actually what was left of our fire extinguisher that just melted." Also, the memory of how black everything appeared covered by charcoal dust has stayed with him.

For Mark and his small practice team, the situation was unbelievable. Nonetheless, they sat down and figured out a way to move forward. The fire occurred on a Friday morning, and by the following Monday, their practice was open again across the road in a vacant space over a pharmacy. They used their strengths of teamwork and hope, working through the weekend to get new computer systems and other essential items. "The show had to go on was kind of the outward message to the world. We're bulletproof."

Unfortunately, even as he appeared resilient to the outer world, his personal "show" didn't go on for weeks afterward. The fire investigators found evidence that suggested the fire was deliberately set. "I had trouble sleeping. I was wondering who did this. I was consumed with why. What'd I do to harm anyone? I had crazy thoughts like, would they come to my house next." He wondered what would happen and grappled with fear and anxiety, and a bit of anger as well. He was also feeling sorry for himself. Worse yet were feelings of guilt about his "poor me" perspective, as he reminded himself that nobody got burned in the fire and that worse things happen to people every single day.

"But I couldn't help how I felt. It caught hold of me for a while, and then I realized that I had to accept what had happened and move on and let go of it. That's one of the best lessons I've ever learned." He learned that he couldn't change what had happened, but he could change how he responded.

Mark embraced this idea of acceptance and leveraged the strengths of gratitude that no one was hurt and forgiveness for the arsonist. Some patients came in to say they knew who set the fire, and the police even charged somebody. "There was all this kind of distraction going on, keeping me thinking about why, but in the end, I had to let go of it."

His years of letting go of negative thoughts and embracing positive attitudes, especially gratitude and self-compassion, paid off. "I now look back on that fire and I'm so grateful for it. That fire taught me so much about resilience and that how you respond to life really matters. Nobody can take that away from us. We all have so much strength within us if we have the courage to tap into that."

Mark believes the fire changed the trajectory of his life. Less than eighteen months later, he built a four-thousand-square-foot facility and took on more support staff. The practice grew rapidly and moved to the Waterford Health Park, where he has been for the last several years. The new setting is beautiful and is his pride. "That spark of possibility and creativity came from the fire. It's something I really understand. Sometimes you have to experience things in life to have that deep learning."

Mark emphasized the power of post-traumatic growth; we get wiser when we make mistakes or experience adverse events by learning from them. "Most people do grow from their traumas. The norm is to grow. People develop a stronger sense of who they are, a stronger sense of spirituality and develop an appreciation for life. I feel so lucky that I went through that [fire], and I can't imagine what my life would have been like if I had not had that fire."

Some of his patients experience a similar change when dealing with a major medical diagnosis, such as cancer; they view life very differently and live in a better, more appreciative way. "While I wouldn't wish ill health on anyone, they can grow from the experience in all sorts of ways, and they wouldn't change that for the world."

A Toolset at Our Inner Core

Character strengths can bolster individuals through tough times and promote growth. This lesson was highlighted through the stories of how I came to adopt my daughter, Margaret's approach to her fellow man in the pandemic, and Mark's blossoming with positivity and gratitude after one of the lowest points in his life.

Growth is more likely to happen when we are empowered with these strength tools. You, too, can take advantage of this lesson with a few straightforward steps. You can identify your signature strengths by taking the VIA survey. You can also keep an eye out for how you successfully handle life's challenges and ask those who know you well to name some positive traits they notice in you. Once you have several strengths identified, keep them top of mind and make a point of applying them every chance you get to achieve your personal and professional goals. You'll find your best self through this fine-tuning process, regardless of the level of traumas you encounter in life.

Key Points

- We can use both our signature strengths and other character strengths to successfully navigate traumas.
- Character strengths, such as forgiveness, gratitude, perseverance, bravery, and hope, can complement other strengths we identify through self-observation and self-discovery.
- We cannot only weather traumas but grow from them.
- Regular application of character strengths in daily life will better prepare us to grow from traumas.
- Although often uninvited, we can choose to embrace traumas as opportunities in our lives to become our best selves.

Reflective Activity: Wellbeing through Trauma

Think back to a traumatic event in your life.

- What was my initial reaction? What were my thoughts and beliefs about what happened? How did I feel?

- How can I embrace self-compassion to move on and grow from the event and the consequences?
- Which character strengths previously helped me not only cope but also move on and do well despite that adversity?
- How did I grow as a result of that experience? What lessons did I learn about myself and my strengths during such times?
- What might I do differently the next time I experience a trauma? How will I support my growth through such challenges?

CHAPTER 11

STRENGTHS IN ACTION

You're off to great places; today is your day. Your mountain is waiting, so get on your way.

—DR. SEUSS

As we implement the activities in the thriving toolkit, we need to think about how we will integrate them into our lives in ways that encourage us to stick with them for the long term. Almost all of us have experienced a time when we knew what we needed to do for our wellbeing, but we didn't achieve the goal or found ourselves easily getting off track. To effectively achieve our wellbeing goals, we can apply several approaches from the health coaching field, including action planning, for the goals we are committed to achieving.

A Cautionary Note

If this process of making new, life-changing habits seems overwhelming, you might consider contacting a health coach. The National Board of Health and Wellness Coaching website (nbhwc.org) can help you find a nationally certified coach who can facilitate your behavior changes. More importantly, if you find yourself hitting a wall, unable to create a positive wellbeing action plan due to significant low moods, stress, or negative emotions, I recommend you reach out to your primary health practitioner or a behavioral health professional to help you manage your mental health. Take care of your immediate needs first. When you feel ready to build habits that enhance resilience and thriving, you can revisit these recommendations.

Action Planning for Your Thriving Habits

The first three toolsets in the toolkit involve three kinds of activities: physical self-care actions, such as eating a healthy diet and being physically active; positive psychology-based activities, such as practicing gratitude; and social interactions, like quality time with family. Using action planning to build these habits into your routine makes sense. But using action planning around the other two toolsets, which are assets you naturally carry—your signature and brain strengths—might not be so obvious. The same approach can be applied to them; the activities involve intentionally using them.

An example from my life includes an action plan to leverage my leadership strength. I regularly volunteer to lead projects and to run for positions in my professional organizations.

I also recently started my own nonprofit organization. This leadership strength extends to my personal life; I stepped in to lead a social group of colleagues when my friend who had been organizing the meetings felt ready to pass the baton. My leadership strength action plan involves a brief monthly check-in and a yearly in-depth review of projects and opportunities.

I also have an action plan to purposefully use my brain strength of extroverted intuition—envisioning various possibilities and patterns in the outer world. My action plan involves taking a moment before each project to reflect on how this brain strength can assist me. Before diving into writing an article, I brainstorm various options to use the content broadly, such as developing an opinion piece for a scientific journal, writing a blog, finding an appropriate podcast to share it, and creating social media posts. Brainstorming this way gets me motivated and excited and propels me to complete the project.

A few of these activities may have jumped out as ones you already fully embrace in your life. Great! Keep it up! You can mentally place those in your toolkit. Or perhaps you have tried one or two in the past, but they did not stick. Reflect on what happened and see how you might want to try again. And if you are not ready to try some of the suggested tools, consider revisiting them later.

If you feel ready to develop an action plan, that's terrific. Let's look at the steps for turning your action goals into habits.

Reviewing Your Thriving Habits and Identifying New Ones

To decide which activities to include in your action plan, first, review what you are already doing. Look at the five sets of tools and assess where you are in each area.

- What are you doing for your self-care? What kind of diet do you eat? Are you as physically active as you want to be? Are you getting enough high-quality sleep? Are you avoiding risky substances?
- What are you doing to grow your capacity to manage stress and boost positive emotions? What activities give you a sense of flow and a sense of meaning and purpose?
- What are the key relationships in your life? What kinds of social support networks do you have, and how are you building positive interactions?
- How do you leverage your signature strengths and other self-identified strengths? What opportunities do you currently have to intentionally use them?
- How do you harness your brain strengths—your ways of both understanding the world and making decisions? Then ask yourself what you are motivated and ready to do. It's okay to set aside some activities for a later time when you feel ready. The goal is to have some early successes.

For each activity you'd like to begin, start with a small step to make sure you'll succeed and build up over time. Ask yourself how willing you are to do the action step on a scale of 0 (not important at all) to 10 (most important thing in your life at this time). Also, rate your change readiness level from 0 (not ready to change) to 10 (very ready to change). By choosing activities that you rate 7 or above, you are more likely to be successful with them (Rollnick, Mason and Butler, 2002).

For example, if you'd like to start a gratitude practice habit, the action plan might look like this, including what you will do, with whom, when, for how long, and how often.

I will sit down with my partner after dinner on Sunday evenings and we'll each share three things for which we are grateful. We'll spend about a half hour on this activity, each of us sharing for fifteen minutes.

Also, set a time by when you would like to achieve your action plan, when you will check on your progress, and how you will know you've succeeded. This approach aligns with setting SMART goals—specific, measurable, attainable, realistic, and time-bound, which are shown to nudge action (Aghera et al., 2018).

When developing action plans, think about what motivates you and the benefits of making the change. Consider possible solutions for potential barriers. This might be a good time to talk to a close friend for support. Perhaps they would like to join you in the journey. Research the information and details you need to help you proceed.

Once you have created your plan, check your confidence level, reassessing that you can achieve it. Where are you on a scale of 0 (not confident at all) to 10 (most confident)? Make sure your confidence with the plan exceeds 6. Dial back the plan if needed. Start with tiny habits and build from there until you achieve your ultimate goal. For example, if you successfully start meditating for ten minutes twice a week, you can steadily increase the amount of time and frequency until you reach your goal of twenty minutes twice a day.

Determine how you'll remind yourself or keep yourself accountable and how you'll evaluate your progress. How often will you check back on your progress, and how will you know you have succeeded? When you have partial successes or come up against challenges, revise your action plan to be certain it's achievable on the next check-in round.

One of the leaders in "persuasive technology," that is, the use of digital devices to nudge behavior, developed a model of B = MAP. Behavior (B) change occurs when the individual's motivation (M), ability (A), and prompts (P) are aligned (Fogg, 2019).

Creating a Relapse Prevention Plan for Your New Thriving Habits

Building positive habits, as with any habit, involves both finding ways to achieve and maintain the activity for the long term. It takes a different set of skills to continue a habit once it is developed. When you are consistently doing your intended activity for a few weeks (Watson, 2020), or even sooner, support yourself to stay on track by developing a relapse prevention plan. The plan guides you to identify when you first get off track, called a lapse, what you will do to get back on track, and to whom you'll reach out for help. This intervention is key before you lose the habit over a significant amount of time and enter a relapse phase. Once in relapse, much more effort may be required to restart.

When I first achieved my goal of walking every afternoon, I developed a relapse prevention plan to help me in case I got off track. When I notice that more than two days have gone by without walking, I ask myself what support I need to walk regularly. If I'm busy with work, I reach out to my partner to nudge me for a brisk walk before dinner.

Achieving and Maintaining Your Action Plans

As you start implementing your action plan, consider ways you can energize yourself to fully achieving and maintaining it. Focus on what is going well. By emphasizing the positive results, even partial successes, we tend to be much more engaged in doing what it takes to reach our goals. We are riding powerful waves of positive emotions. That's why celebrating all successes, big and small, represents an essential element of action planning.

Reach out to an accountability buddy—a family member or friend with whom you can share your vision of success. They cannot only help keep you accountable by reminding you of your goal but also enthusiastically cheer you on and celebrate your successes with you. The more you think about and talk about change and the more detailed your vision of a positive future of thriving through your new habits, the more likely you will make it a reality.

Consider regularly reflecting on your action plan or keeping a journal. Describe the best parts of your experiences and brainstorm solutions to challenges that make you optimistic about overcoming them. Identify your most powerful motivators and the strengths you used to achieve your progress. Explain how this new way of being and living aligns with your core values. List the people, resources, and apps that have been the greatest support for you. Make the best use of them and reach for additional supports as needed.

Along the path of creating habits, you may find yourself experiencing doubts and thinking unsupportive thoughts. Many resources from the long-standing field of cognitive behavioral therapy reinforce how we can pay attention to our self-talk and reframe it if it is not productive. For example, an individual who has set a plan to write in a gratitude practice journal weekly may find herself muttering, "I'll never have the time because weekdays are busy with work and weekends are filled with chores." Through self-awareness of these thoughts, she can stop and reframe them in a more supportive way: "This goal is important to me, and I can set aside just a few minutes on Sunday evenings, which tend to be less busy" (Claiborn and Pedrick, 2001).

Reinforcing Your Action Plans

As you are learning and adapting to your thriving activities, take advantage of what you have discovered about how you learn best. Purposefully recalling positive memories while engaging in the desired behavior can trigger positive emotions, driving an unconscious motivation to do the behavior again and again (Kok et al., 2013).

For example, if your goal is to start a gratitude practice, you might write down your commitment on a piece of paper and place it on your refrigerator. After you do the gratitude practice and are swimming in positive emotions, look at the note and touch the refrigerator. Then every time you open the refrigerator, the note may serve not only as a reminder but also as a trigger of those positive emotions, reinforcing your plan.

As you consider your plan for each strength toolset, create a compelling vision of engaging with those tools. Paint a picture in your mind of what you will look like doing that activity, how you will feel having achieved that level of wellness and thriving, and what kind of a person you will become as a result of the ongoing application of the tools in the thriving toolkit. This approach from positive psychology will stir up those important positive emotions.

Author's Thriving Tools

You might be wondering how I developed my action plans as a lifestyle medicine physician and positive psychology enthusiast. Over the years, I have gone through a "trial and correction" process with a variety of self-care and positive activity habits, as well as using my signature and brain strengths. I keep a list of the habits that have worked for me on my phone and update the list at least every year.

When I started, I had to make adjustments every few weeks and learned early on that I was more successful when I wrote down my action steps and discussed them with a friend. I've also discovered that the best time to revisit my action plans is when I am feeling good and feel the energy to recommit to my wellbeing. I cement in my memory those positive emotions and relive them during times when I feel challenged to stay on track.

Through this process, I now have some favorite wellbeing habits. I take walks each day and eat a colorful and delicious whole-food plant-based diet. I especially enjoy tomatoes and cucumbers on whole wheat with balsamic reduction dressing. And ripe raspberries are definitely the most decadent dessert flavor for me!

I enjoy engaging fully with my hobbies, especially drawing and painting—a satisfying and mindful activity that makes the rest of the world melt away. I look forward to regular heartfelt chats with close friends, as well as participating in two women's support groups. I am always cognizant of the meaningful moments I experience in assisting both my daughter and my mother with their needs and relish the times we laugh together. Applying these lifestyle approaches contributes immensely to my sense of vitality.

I make a point of using my signature strengths, especially leadership and perseverance and my brain strength of extroverted intuition—envisioning many new possibilities for solutions and actions. I am leveraging these strengths to support myself through the hard work of establishing a new nonprofit organization to promote positive psychology in health care. I find it invigorating to envision what we can accomplish together and to brainstorm options for engaging health practitioners and systems in this exciting endeavor.

During my regular life review, I harness my brain strength to see the patterns of my life—where I have been, where I am headed, and how what I am doing fits with my life goals to give me a sense of meaning and accomplishment. Enhancing this review through a positive psychology lens allows me to readily identify patterns of what is going well in my friendships, professional endeavors, and my painting and travel hobbies.

I've also discovered that I can apply my brain strength in my art by visualizing new paintings. This approach can quickly take me into a world of shelter from the storm. I can spend hours immersed in the possibilities of color, style, and shape. After emerging from the experience, I notice myself smiling heartily. At times, I even feel an extra bolt of energy and a sense of aliveness. My whole body straightens with enthusiasm, and at the same time, a calm comes over me.

Of course, like everyone, I sometimes run into snags in keeping up with my thriving activities. When I face major deadlines and work projects that have piled on at the same time, I can find myself slacking on my walking routine and not visiting friends as often as I like. When I notice this happening, I make a point of shortening the time I spend on these activities. In this way, I maintain my habits while freeing up some additional time for my work. As soon as the deadlines are met, I enjoy reinvigorating my full action plan.

I hope the strategies summarized here from the health coaching and positive psychology fields encourage you to develop your vision and plan for this kind of thriving. Implementing and fully embracing these habits will serve you well and hoist you up on the road of life. Choose what you are ready to do, set an action plan with small achievable steps leading to your ultimate goals, use your signature, brain and other strengths, evaluate your progress, celebrate successes—even partial ones, incite positive emotions along the way, and get the support and assistance you need.

Through these wellbeing action planning steps, you are very likely to succeed!

Key Points
- Develop your self-care and positive and social activities into action plans.
- Harness signature and brain strengths, your innate qualities, by developing action plans for intentionally and regularly using them.

- Review your current thriving activities and check to see which ones need adjusting and which new ones you feel ready to incorporate into your lifestyle.
- Create specific action plans that will help you develop new thriving habits. Make sure that you are confident you can achieve them. If not, adjust the planned action steps to smaller ones to ensure success.
- Develop relapse prevention plans for the times when you notice you are off track so that you can decide how you'll get back in the groove.
- Look for ways to boost positive emotions when engaged in these activities.
- Make a point of reliving those positive feelings to drive you to do the activities again and again.
- Use other strategies that have helped you build habits in the past. Examples include visualizing a positive future if you succeed and journaling about your progress toward your goals.
- Always celebrate your successes, even partial ones, and savor those good feelings.

Reflective Activity and Checklist of Your *Strengths in the Mirror* Takeaways

- What are my major takeaways from this book?
- What tools will I include in my thriving toolkit?
- What specific strengths will I rely on as my key pillars for thriving?
- What is my next action step on the road to enhanced wellbeing and flourishing?

EPILOGUE

THRIVING NOW AND TOMORROW

Our *Strengths in the Mirror* journey highlighted tools for thriving based on the fields of lifestyle medicine and positive psychology. With these tools, you can access the power that emanates from the reciprocal and reinforcing relationship of healthy habits and positive emotions. You can also craft an approach that purposefully embraces your signature and brain strengths.

We need to fine-tune our strengths to make the most of them in the face of growing challenges in our modern, evolving society. The COVID-19 pandemic, sociopolitical conflicts, and other unsettling events have led to increasing levels of stress. That increased stress can lead to unhealthy lifestyles, poor mental health, and substance misuse. High social media use, bordering on and becoming an addiction for some, is contributing to depression and anxiety and distracts from positive habits. Moreover, the percent of individuals feeling socially isolated and lonely has risen significantly and is now a looming public health crisis.

Regular positive psychology and healthy practices can lead to positive health that bolsters our capacity to grow even in adversity. Based on ancient wisdom and modern science, the core truths about what supports and builds our wellbeing resonate through the stories and messages shared by health professionals. I feel privileged that a few of them have graciously shared their stories with us. I find inspiration from their wise insights and encouraging words. I hope you have too.

Before reading this book, you were likely engaging in some self-care activities that boost both physical and emotional health. Perhaps our journey has nudged you to view a healthy lifestyle through a wider lens to include routine positive psychology habits and the application of your character and brain strengths, along with a healthy diet, physical activity, and sleep.

What Will You Do Now to Boost Your Thriving?

So what's in your toolkit? Have you considered making changes to your daily thriving practices? How will you bring together healthy lifestyles, positive habits, and your innate personal strengths in ways that will serve you best? Create your action plan, check your progress, and celebrate your successes.

The reciprocal, reinforcing link between these activities might not always be highlighted in medicine. Yet I hope now you see how this link lies at the core of your total wellbeing. Physical, mental, emotional, social, spiritual, and positive health are all intertwined.

When we catch ourselves struggling with what we "should do" to be healthy, we might look to build actions that bring us a sense of vitality and life satisfaction, and then the rest may fall into place. Your medical practitioner can and should encourage and support you in incorporating these activities into your healthy lifestyle maintenance and treatment approaches.

Plan your day with delicious plant-based meals, invigorating physical movement, and refreshing sleep, and look for and savor the positive emotions. Do what leads to a state of flow, interact positively with others, and engage in activities that give you a sense of meaning and accomplishment. Those positive feelings can drive you to continue healthy habits and lead to building additional resources in an upward spiral of positive changes.

Positive changes can be further advanced when you regularly use character strengths to enhance your self-efficacy and preparedness for any situation. Purposefully turn to your brain strengths to achieve your goals more easily and allow them to energize you. Along with other self-identified strengths, you can build up your internal "muscles" for thriving.

A few health behaviorists I know sometimes smile and joke that the best health behaviors are the ones people will do. Indeed! Identify the activities that work well for you and weave them into your routine. The more well-practiced and versatile the tools in your toolkit, the more you will feel ready for life's demands and joys while growing into your best self.

When I give presentations, I'm often asked if I had to choose only one tool to start, which would it be. My answer is positive social connections. If you do nothing else, increase positive interactions with friends and family and even brief authentic exchanges with strangers or acquaintances. High-quality connections in which we experience synchronous positive emotions trigger strong physiologic, as well as psychologic, benefits—leading to happiness and physical health. Although the definitive verdict is out about the impact of using social media often, it'd be prudent to use it sparingly. Make a point of getting together in person.

A Closing Inspiration

I'd like to close with another story, this one from Retired Brigadier General Rhonda Cornum. Her incredible story of leaving her teenage daughter to serve as a flight surgeon in the Gulf War and her experience as a POW after being shot down are described in her book, *She Went to War*. I've had the pleasure of volunteering with her in the International Positive Psychology Association and on our Global Positive Health Institute Advisory Council, where I noticed her "can-do," matter-of-fact approach to our projects. Her interest in working to promote positive psychology is no surprise, as one can immediately notice her natural inclination to embrace many of its tools. I confirmed this in a recent chat with her.

In Rhonda's down-to-earth style, she shared a story that highlights one of her secret positive psychology weapons in day-to-day life, as well as during small or large traumatic events. Let's see if you can quickly spot it. "I was driving my truck with a horse trailer behind me. I was trying to get them (the horses) to the vet and still get to work on time, so I was going a little fast." At a curve in the road, her truck rolled down a hill; fortunately, her trailer came up off the ball in the back.

She shared what happened and the thoughts going through her mind in those moments. "Eventually, my truck stopped at the bottom of the hill, and I'm not dead. It's kind of squashed, but I'm short, so I could see out what's left of the window, and I saw my trailer. I said to myself, 'Oh, good, the horses probably aren't hurt.' Next, I said, 'I'm glad I was wearing my seatbelt; if I had not been wearing my seatbelt, my head would have been out the window, and it would have been like a squashed melon.' The third thing I said to myself was, 'I'm so glad I didn't bring the dog; he would have gotten thrown out of the truck.'" She then crawled out the broken window, noticed that she wasn't hurt, and felt very lucky.

She called the police, notified the people expecting her, made arrangements to be picked up, and went about her day. "It could have been a traumatic experience. But it wasn't. It was just inconvenient." Focusing on the good things and gratitude helped her through that event. She emphasizes it as a steady aspect of her life. "Every minute, you find something to be grateful for. No matter how bad it is, it could have been worse. The glass is half full instead of half empty."

As you follow this kind of thriving path that embraces a healthy lifestyle and a positive approach to life, you are building your capacity to turn to the most reliable resource at your disposal—yourself. Look in the mirror; the strengths that comprise your best self are staring back. Use them and you'll very likely find yourself thriving now and tomorrow.

PART 4

RESOURCES

IDENTIFYING BRAIN STRENGTHS

What's Your Personality Type?

To identify your type, you can take the Myers-Briggs Type Indicator questionnaire, a proprietary questionnaire that can be accessed through a certified counselor. But even this well-studied questionnaire will only give you an estimate of your best-fit type.

Your mood, a recent event or interaction, or your environment can predispose you to provide answers that are not true to your type. That is why it is advisable to read the descriptions and think about which one fits you best based on what you already know about yourself from life experience.

Continue to observe yourself in different circumstances until you are confident you have identified the type that best fits you. *Type Talk* by Otto Kroeger and Janet M. Thuesen is an example of a resource that gives a succinct overview of each type and will broaden your understanding of personality type.

For the purpose of this thriving toolkit, it's more important to determine what brain strengths you believe fit you best based on the checklist and chart below and self-observation of how you gather information and make decisions. You can learn to refine those mental processes to your thriving advantage.

Personality Type Questionnaire

Select one option in each group. Even if you identify with both options, choose the one you tend to rely on most often or one to which you are more strongly drawn. When you are in a situation that requires you to think or act quickly which would you likely think or do? (Lianov, 2013).

Source of Energy When Interacting with the Outer versus Inner World

Extroversion (E):

Someone who prefers extroversion:

- Is drawn to and derives energy from the outer world and interacting with others
- Prefers to talk to figure things out and to communicate
- Is in tune with the outside environment
- Energized by being sociable and by open discussions
- Has a variety of interests and prefers to know many people
- Reflects after speaks

OR

Introversion (I):

- *Focuses on the inner world and gets energy from reflection on memories and feelings and inward attention*
- *Prefers to figure things out by inwardly reflecting*
- *Tends to be private and reveal selected things*
- *Has in-depth interests and prefers knowing a few people well*
- *Prefers to think before speaking*
- *Enjoys and is energized by spending time alone*

What is your source of energy? E or I?

Taking in Information

Sensing (S):

- *Focuses on gathering tangible information and observing specifics in the outside environment*
- *Is drawn to concrete facts*
- *Uses practical applications to understand ideas*
- *Learns by doing step-by-step*
- *Prefers direct experience*
- *Focuses on the actual situation and present reality*

OR

iNtuition (N):

- *Gathers information by seeing the big picture, connections, patterns, and relationships*
- *Likes to consider future possibilities*
- *Prefers to figure out meanings behind patterns and information*
- *Focuses on ideas first before putting them into practice*
- *Trusts insights or hunches*
- *Needs to see the big picture and then remember and learn the facts*

How do you prefer to take information from the world? S or N?

Decision Making

Thinking (T):

- *Looks at the logic of each option to make a decision*
- *Is drawn to critique the situation; identifies the pros and cons and the costs and benefits*
- *Tends to be analytical*
- *Seeks fairness by making sure everyone is treated equally*
- *Prefers to apply objective criteria*
- *Looks at cause and effect*
- *Is usually swayed by logic*

OR

Feeling (F):

- *Considers what is important to self and others and makes decisions based on values*
- *Is energized by supporting others and making sure others feel appreciated*
- *First considers the impact of decisions on others*
- *Is drawn to harmonious situations and is uncomfortable with disagreements*
- *Places highest importance on personal values*
- *Is seen as compassionate, empathetic, and personal*

How do you tend to make decisions? T or F?

Arranging the Outer World

Judging (J):

- *Prefers to have his life planned and orderly*
- *Is drawn to come to closure as soon as possible*
- *Prefers to have things decided and settled*
- *Is drawn to a schedule, with one project completed before the next is begun*
- *Likes to feel things are being done in a planned way*
- *Prefers life to be organized and planned*
- *Is comfortable with routine*

OR

Perceiving:

- *Is drawn to flexibility and being spontaneous, keeping things open-ended*
- *Likes to be open to make a change*
- *Is energized by last-minute pressure*
- *Is adaptable, flexible*
- *Enjoys multiple projects at the same time*
- *Is comfortable improvising*

How do you prefer to have the outer world arranged? J or P?

What Are Your Brain Strengths?

Now that you have identified an estimate of your personality type, let's learn what your type indicates about ways you learn from the world and what influences your decisions. Two groups of mental processes form the core of the personality framework. One group describes four ways an individual can gather information about the world, and another group describes four ways an individual can make decisions.

Each personality type has a preferred mental process for information gathering and decision-making. One of these two is dominant, and the other auxiliary. I refer to them in this book as brain strengths. We use the other six mental processes as needed but with less ease, requiring more attention and energy.

The chart below lists the brain strengths—dominant and auxiliary mental processes—of each type (Lianov, 2013).

Dominant and Auxiliary Mental Processes of Each Personality Type

ISTJ *Dominant:* Introverted sensing *Auxiliary* Extroverted thinking	**ISFJ** *Dominant:* Introverted sensing *Auxiliary:* Extroverted feeling	**INFJ** *Dominant:* Introverted intuition *Auxiliary:* Extroverted feeling	**INTJ** *Dominant:* Introverted intuition *Auxiliary:* Extroverted thinking
ISTP *Dominant:* Introverted thinking *Auxiliary:* Extroverted sensing	**ISFP** *Dominant:* Introverted feeling *Auxiliary:* Extroverted sensing	**INFP** *Dominant:* Introverted feeling *Auxiliary:* Extroverted intuition	**INTP** *Dominant:* Introverted thinking *Auxiliary:* Extroverted intuition
ESTP *Dominant:* Extroverted sensing *Auxiliary:* Introverted thinking	**ESFP** *Dominant:* Extroverted sensing *Auxiliary:* Introverted feeling	**ENFP** *Dominant:* Extroverted intuition *Auxiliary:* Introverted feeling	**ENTP** *Dominant:* Extroverted intuition *Auxiliary:* Introverted thinking
ESTJ *Dominant:* Extroverted thinking *Auxiliary:* Introverted sensing	**ESFJ** *Dominant:* Extroverted feeling *Auxiliary:* Introverted sensing	**ENFJ** *Dominant:* Extroverted feeling *Auxiliary:* Introverted intuition	**ENTJ** *Dominant:* Extroverted thinking *Auxiliary:* Introverted intuition

ADDITIONAL GUIDANCE AND TOOLS

Action for Happiness: https://www.actionforhappiness.org
American College of Lifestyle Medicine:
  https://www.lifestylemedicine.org
Benson-Henry Institute for Mind Body Medicine:
  https://bensonhenryinstitute.org/
Global Positive Health Institute, Inc.: https://positivehealth.world
Greater Good Science Center: http://greatergood.berkeley.edu/
Greater Good in Action: http://ggia.berkeley.edu/
My Happy Avatar site and link to app:
  http://www.myhappyavatar.com/
International Positive Psychology Association:
  https://www.ippanetwork.org/
Lee Kum Sheung (Harvard). Center for Health and Happiness, Harvard TH Chan School of Public Health:
  https://www.hsph.harvard.edu/health-happiness
Masters in Applied Positive Psychology Program:
  https://www.sas.upenn.edu/lps/graduate/mapp
Mayo Clinic Healthy Living Program:
  https://healthyliving.mayoclinic.org

Science of Wellbeing Course: https://www.cousera.org/learn/the-science-of-wellbeing

Personality Types, app with brief Myers-Briggs questionnaire by Radiance House (Dario Nardi).

Positive Psychology Center, University of Pennsylvania: https://www.ppc.sas.upenn.edu

Stanford University—Center for Compassion and Altruism Research and Education: https://ccare.stanford.edu/

The Myers & Briggs Foundation: https://www.myersbriggs.org/; Take the MBTI at: https://www.myersbriggs.org/my-mbti-personality-type/take-the-mbti-instrument

The Wholebeing Institute: https://wholebeinginstitute.com/

Society of Behavioral Medicine: https://www.sbm.org/

VIA Institute on Character Survey—Character Strengths: http://www.viacharacter.org/

Yale University—Center for Emotional Intelligence: https://www.ei.yale.edu

ACKNOWLEDGMENTS

The process of writing and publishing a book is a huge endeavor and requires much support. I'd like to call out the many individuals who helped make this dream come true.

I'm immensely grateful to Christin Collins, who suggested I join Eric Koester's group of students in the fall of 2020. That powerful encouragement began this incredible journey. Thank you, Eric Koester, for all the wisdom and guidance and to the team at New Degree Press. I've learned so much and have grown through the experience.

My heartfelt thanks go to the colleagues and friends who agreed to be interviewed and to share their inspirational stories full of wisdom and practical advice: Kaylan Baban, Carrie Barron, Rhonda Cornum, Margaret Moore, Dario Nardi, Ryan Niemiec, Robin Ortiz, Parneet Pal, Dani Pere, and Mark Rowe. You provided the soul of this book!

I give my sincere gratitude to Karen Siener, Simon Matthews, and Joe Raphael, who provided invaluable guidance and editing assistance.

Many thanks to the members of my Author's Circle, who contributed to the book campaign and came along on this book journey. Your support made it so much more worthwhile:

Alicia Abels, Anjana Aggarwal, Melyssa Allen, Carol Alley, Anita Balan, Patti Barker, Carrie Barron, Sharon Bergquist, Alison Breen, Madeline Brady, Nan Clark, Cate Collings, Christin Collins, Kristen Collins, Susana Crispin, Maria Crompton, Ingrid Edshteyn, Susan Fellman, Patricia Foster, Kelly Freeman, Lew Fulton, Karen Garman, Prachi Garodia, Marianne Hernandez, Jeff Hougen, Kara Houston, Natalie Hsu, Manika Jain, Anitha Kankar, Scott Kashman, Andrea Klemes, Eric Koester, Kristina Leventhal, Simon Matthews, Sam McClellan, Gia Merlo, Suzen Moeller, Ifeoma Monye, Margaret Moore, Lou Morris, Joanne Murphy, Tiffany Nguyen, Kay Nicholas, Ike Nnene, Elaine O'Brien, Joan O'Connor, Jane Oh, Kimmie Ouchi, Parneet Pal, Erin Phillips, Dee Prince, Joe Raphael, Jessica Repa, Jennifer Rooke, Mark Rowe, Deepa Sannidhi, Nancy and Bob Schlag, Pamela Schmidt, Iris Schrijver, Karen Siener, Karen Struder, Michele Suhie, Rebecca Teng, Maria and Mark Tebbutt, Michelle Tollefson, Cheryl True, Dorothy Woody, and Eileen Yamada.

This book occupied much of my attention and time for nearly a year. Heartfelt gratitude to my family for enduring and cheerleading the process! Special thanks to my daughter Lorelei Bergerson, my mother Tania Lianov, and my dear Lew Fulton.

Thank you, future readers! I wish you love, happiness, health, success, and a sense of vitality. Squeeze the best from life and spread the pearls of inspiration, wisdom, and positive nudges with friends, family, and our global community.

Happy, healthy regards always!

In the spirit of powerful gratitude and in the fun words of Dr. Seuss, I feel "muchly much-much" lucky, dear readers, colleagues, and friends, for sharing life with you! You contribute to my happiness. I leave you with this inspiration:

Let us be grateful to the people who make us happy; they are the charming gardeners who make our souls blossom.

—MARCEL PROUST

APPENDIX

Introduction

Boehm, Julia K, Sonja Lyubomirsky, and Kennon M. Sheldon. "A Longitudinal Experimental Study Comparing the Effectiveness of Happiness-Enhancing Strategies in Anglo Americans and Asian Americans." *Cognition and Emotion* 2, no. 7 (2011): 1263-72. https://doi.org/10.1080/02699931.2010.541227.

Diener, Ed and Louise Tay. "Needs and Subjective Wellbeing Around the World." *Journal of Personality and Social Psychology* 101 no. 2 (2011): 354-365. https://doi.org/10.1037/a0023779.

Emmons, Robert A, and Michael E. McCullough. "Counting Blessings Versus Burdens: Experimental Studies of Gratitude and Subjective Wellbeing." *Journal of Personality and Social Psychology* 84, no. 2 (2003): 377-389. https://doi.org/10.1037/0022-3514.84.2.377.

Hendriks, Ton, Marijke Schotanus-Dijkstra, Aabidien Hassankhan, Joop de Jong, and Ernst Bohlmeijer. "The efficacy of multi-component Positive Psychology Interventions: A systematic review and meta-analysis of Randomized Controlled

Trials." *Journal of Happiness Studies* 21 (2020): 357-390. https://doi.org/10.1007/s10902-019-00082-1.

Layous, Kristin, Huyunjung Lee, Incheol Choi, and Sonja Lyubomirsky. "Culture Matters When Designing a Successful Happiness-Increasing Activity: A Comparison of the United States and South Korea." *Journal of Cross-Cultural Psychology* 44 no. 8 (2013): 1294-1303. https://doi.org/10.1177/0022022113487591.

Lianov, Liana. *Roots of Positive Change, Optimizing Healthcare with Positive Psychology.* Fair Oaks, CA: Healthtype LLC in collaboration with the American College of Lifestyle Medicine, 2019.

Nelson-Coffey, S. Katherine, Megan M Fritz, Sonja Lyubomirsky, and Steve W Cole. "Kindness in the Blood: A Randomized Controlled Trial of the Gene Regulatory Impact of Prosocial Behavior." *Psychoneuroendocrinology* 81 (2017): 8-13. https://doi.org/10.1016/j.psyneuen.2017.03.025.

Sandstrom, Gillian M, and Elizabeth W. Dunn. "Social Interactions and Wellbeing: The Surprising Power of Weak Ties." *Personality and Social Psychology Bulletin* 40(2014): 910-922. https://doi.org/10.1177/0146167214529799.

Taleb, Nassim Nicholas. *Antifragile: Things that Gain from Disorder.* New York, NY: Random House Publishing Group, 2014.

Chapter 1: How We Got Here

American College of Lifestyle Medicine. Accessed June 12, 2021. https://www.lifestylemedicine.org.

American Psychological Association. "Stress in America™ 2020, A National Mental Health Crisis." Accessed June 23, 2021. https://www.apa.org/news/press/releases/stress/2020/report-october.

Gable, Shelly L, and Jonathan Haidt. "What (and Why) Is Positive Psychology?" *Review of General Psychology* 9, no. 2 (2005): 103-110. https://doi.org/10.1037/1089-2680.9.2.103.

Heath, Chip, and Dan Heath. *Switch: How to Change Things When Change is Hard*. New York, NY: Crown Business, 2010.

Jacka, Felice N, Adrienne O'Neil, Rachel Opie, Catherine Itsiopoulos, Sue Cotton, Mohammedreza Mohebbi, David Castel, Saraj Dasj, Catherine Mihalopoulos, Mary Lou Chatterton, Laima Brazionis, Olivia M Dean, Allison M Hodge, and Michael Berk. "A Randomized Controlled Trial of Dietary Improvement for Adults with Major Depression (the 'SMILES' Trial)." *BMC Medicine* 15, no. 1 (2017): 23. https://doi.org/10.1186/s12916-017-0791-y.

Kok, Bethany E, Kimberly A Coffey, Michael A Cohn, Lahnna I Catalino, Tanya Vacharklksemusk, Sara B Algoe, Mary Brantley, and Barbara Fredrickson. "How Positive Emotions Build Physical Health: Perceived Positive Social Connections Account for the Upward Spiral Between Positive Emotions and Vagal Tone." *Psychological Science* 24 (2013): 1123-1132. https://doi.org/10.1177/0956797612470827.

Lianov, Liana, and Mark Johnson. "Physician Competencies for Prescribing Lifestyle Medicine." *Journal of the American Medical Association* 304, no. 2 (2010): 202-203.

Lianov, Liana. *My Happy Avatar, Use Our Mobile Devise and Personality to Transform Your Health*. Fair Oaks, CA: HealthType LLC, 2013.

Lianov, Liana, *Roots of Positive Change, Optimizing Health Care with Positive Psychology*. Fair Oaks, CA: HealthType LLC with the American College of Lifestyle Medicine, 2019.

Kushlev, Kostadin, Samantha J Heintzelman, Lesley D Lutes, Derrick Wirtz, Jacqueline M Kanippayoor, Damian Leitner, and Ed Diener. "Does Happiness Improve Health? Evidence from a Randomized Controlled Trial." *Psychological Science* 31, no. 7 (2020): 807-821. https://doi.org/10.1177/0956797620919673.

Morton, Darren. "Healthy Lifestyle Practices and Emotional Wellbeing." In *Roots of Positive Change, Optimizing Health Care with Positive Psychology* edited by Liana Lianov. Fair Oaks, CA: HealthType LLC, 2019.

Nardi, Dario. *Neuroscience of Personality, Brain Savvy Insights for All Types of People.* Los Angeles, CA: Radiance House, 2011.

Ornish, Dean. *Love and Survival. 8 Pathways to Intimacy and Health.* New York, NY: Harper Perennial, Harper Collins Publishers, 1998.

Ornish, Dean, SE Brown, JH Billings, LW Scherwitz, WT Armstrong, TA Ports, SM McLanahan, RL Kirkeeide, KL Gould, and RJ Brand. "Can Lifestyle Changes Reverse Coronary Heart Disease? The Lifestyle Heart Trial." *Lancet* 336(1990): 129-33. https://doi.org/10.1016/0140-6736(90)91656-U.

TEDx Talks. "The Healing Power of Love and Intimacy." Aug 7, 2019. Video 15:31. https://www.ted.com/talks/dean_ornish_the_healing_power_of_love_intimacy.

Seligman, Martin, and Mihalyi Cziksentmihalyi. "Positive Psychology: An Introduction." *American Psychologist* 55 (2000): 5-14. https://doi.org/10.1037/0003-066x.55.1.5.

Seligman, Martin EP. "Positive Health." *Applied. Psychology* 57, no. s1 (2008): 3-18. https://doi.org/10.1111/j.1464-0597.2008.00351.x.

Virtues in Action Institute on Character. Accessed June 23, 2021. https://viacharacter.org.

Van Cappellen, Patty, Elise L Rice, Lahnna I Catalino, and Barbara Fredrickson. "Positive Affective Processes Underlie Positive Health Behavior Change." *Psychology and Health* 33, no. 1 (2018): 77-97. https://doi.org/10.1080/08870446.2017.1320798.

Waters, Lea, Sata B Algoe, Jane Dutton, Robert Emmons, Barbara L Fredrickson, Emily Heaphy, Judith T Moskowitz, Kristen Neff,

Ryan Niemiec, Cynthia Pury, and Michael Steger. "Positive Psychology in a Pandemic: Buffering, Bolstering, and Building Mental Health." *The Journal of Positive Psychology*. February 9, 2021. https://doi.org/10.1080/17439760.2021.1871945.

Chapter 2: Why Now?

Abramson, Ashley. "Substance Use during the Pandemic. Opioid and Stimulant Use is on the Rise—How Psychologists and Other Clinicians Help a Greater Number of Patients Struggling With Drug Use?" American Psychological Association. *Monitor on Psychology* 52, no. 2 (2021): 22. https://www.apa.org/monitor/2021/03/substance-use-pandemic.

American Psychological Association. "Stress in America™ 2020, A National Mental Health Crisis." Accessed June 23, 2021. https://www.apa.org/news/press/releases/stress/2020/report-october.

Cooney, Gary M, Kerry Dwan, Carolyn A Greig, Debbie A Lawlor, Jane Rimer, Fiona R Waugh, Marion McMurdo, and Gilliam E Mead. "Exercise for Depression (Review)." *The Cochrane Database Systematic Reviews* 9 (2013): CD004366. https://doi.org/10.1002/14651858.CD004366.pub6.

Butler Center for Research. "Applications of Positive Psychology to Substance Use Disorder." (May 2017). https://www.hazeldenbettyford.org/education/bcr/addiction-research/positive-psychology-ru-517.

Frates, Beth, Jonathan P Bonnet, Richard Joseph, and James A Peterson. *Lifestyle Medicine Handbook, An Introduction to the Power of Health Habits*. Monterey, CA: Healthy Living.

Harvard Health Letter. "Blue light has a dark side." Harvard Health Publishing, Harvard Medical School. July 7, 2020.

http://www.health.harvard.edu/staying-healthy/blue-light-has-a-dark-side.

Holt-Lunstad, Julianne. "Social isolation and health." Health Affairs Health Policy Brief," June 22, 2020. https://doi.org/10.1377/hpb20200622.253235.

Karim, Fazida, Azeezat A Oyewande, Lamis F Abdalla, Reem Chaudhry Ehsanullah, and Safeera Khan. "Social Media Use and Its Connection to Mental Health: A Systematic Review." *Cureus* 12, no. 6 (2020): e8627. https://doi.org/10.7759/cureus.8627.

Kennedy, Gail. "Stress in America 2021: Pandemic Stress One Year On." American Psychological Association. March 15, 2021. https://www.pacesconnection.com/blog/stress-in-america-2021-pandemic-stress-one-year-on-apa-org.

Kenney, Caitlin M. "VA's Whole Health Program for Veterans Shows Drop in Opioid Use." Stars & Stripes. March 12, 2021. https://www.stripes.com/news/us/va-s-whole-health-program-for-veterans-shows-drop-in-opioid-use-1.665602.

Substance Abuse and Mental Health Services Administration (SAHMSA) Key Substance Use and Mental Health Indicators in the United States: Results from the 2019 National Survey on Drug Use and Health. (September 2020). https://www.samhsa.gov/data/sites/default/files/reports/rpt29393/2019NSDUHFFRPD-FWHTML/2019NSDUHFFR1PDFW090120.pdf.

Krentzman, Amy R. "Review of the Application of Positive Psychology to Substance Use, Addiction, and Recovery Research." *Psychology of Addictive Behaviors: Journal of the Society of Psychologists in Addictive Behaviors* 27, no. 1 (2013): 151-165. https://doi.org/10.1037/a0029897.

Lange, David. "Physical Activity—Statistics & Facts." *Statista*. March 16, 2021. https://www.statista.com/topics/1749/physical-activity/.

Lin, Liu Yi, James E Sidani, Ariel Shensa, Ana Radovic, Elizabeth Miller, Jason B Colditz, Beth L Hoffman, Leila M Giles, and Brian M Primack. "Association between Social Media Use and Depression among US young adults." *Depression and Anxiety* 33, no. 4 (2016): 323-331. https://doi.org/10.1002/da.22466.

Major, Brett C, Khoa D Le Nguyen, Kristjen Lundberg, and Barbara Fredrickson. "Wellbeing Correlates of Perceived Positivity Resonance: Evidence from Trait and Episode-Level Assessments." *Personality and Social Psychology Bulletin* 44, no. 12 (2018): 1631-1647. https://doi.org/10.1177/0146167218771324.

Martino, Jessica, Pegg, Jennifer, and Elizabeth Pegg Frates. "The Connection Prescription: Using the Power of Social Interactions and the Deep Desire for Connectedness to Empower Health and wellness." *American Journal of Lifestyle Medicine* 11, no. 6 (2017): 466-475. https://doi.org/10.1177/1559827615608788.

McGinty, Emma E, Rachel Presskreischer, Hahrie Han, and Colleen L Barry. "Psychological Distress and Loneliness Reported by US adults in 2018 and April 2020." *Journal of the American Medical Association* 324, no. 1 (2020): 93-94. https://doi.org/10.1001/jama.2020.9740.

Mental Health America. 2021 State of Mental Health in America. https://www.mhanational.org/research-reports/2021-state-mental-health-america.

Moore, Latetia V, Kevin W Dodd, Francis E Thompson, Kirsten A Grimm, Sonia A Kim, and Kelley S Scanlon. "Using Behavioral Risk Factor Surveillance System Data to Estimate the Percent of the Population Meeting USDA Food Patterns Fruit and Vegetable Intake Recommendations." *American Journal of Epidemiology* 181, no. 12 (2015): 979-988. https://doi.org/10.1093/aje/kwu461.

Mujcic, Redzo, and Andrew J Oswald. "Evolution of Wellbeing and Happiness after Increases in Consumption of Fruit and

Vegetables." *American Journal of Public Health* 106, no. 8 (2016): 1504-10. https://doi.org/10.2105/AJPH.2016.303260.

Novatoney, Amy. "The Risks of Social Isolation." *American Psychological Association. Monitor in Psychology* 50, no. 5 (May 2019): 32. https://www.apa.org/monitor/2019/05/ce-corner-isolation.

Sandstrom, Gillian M, and Elizabeth W. Dunn. "Social Interactions and Wellbeing: The Surprising Power of Weak Ties." *Personality and Social Psychology Bulletin* 40 (2014): 910-922. https://doi.org/10.1177/0146167214529799.

Seabrook, Elizabeth M, Margaret L Kern, and Nikki S Rickard. "Social Networking Sites, Depression, and Anxiety: A Systemic Review." *JMIR Mental Health* 3, no. 4 (2016): e50. https://doi.org/10.2196/mental.5842.

Waters, Lea, Sara B Algoe, Jane Dutton, Robert Emmons, Barbara L Fredrickson, Emily Heaphy, Judith T Moskowitz, Kristin Neff, Kristin, Ryan Niemiec, Cynthia Pury, and Michael Steger. "Positive Psychology in a Pandemic: Buffering, Bolstering, and Building Mental Health." *The Journal of Positive Psychology*. February 9, 2021. https://doi.org/10.1080/17439760.2021.1871945.

White, Bonnie A, Caroline C Horwath, and Tamlin S Cooner. "Many Apples a Day Keep the Blues Away—Daily Experiences of Negative and Positive Affect and Food Consumption in Young Adults." *British Journal of Health Psychology* 18, no. 4 (2013): 782-798. https://doi.org/10.1111/bjhp.12021.

Chapter 3: Strengths We Create

Barnes, LL, CF Mendes de Leon, RS Wilson, JL Bienias, and DA Evans. "Social Resources and Cognitive Decline in a Population of Older African Americans and Whites." *Neu-*

rology 63, no. 12 (2004): 2322-26. https://doi.org/10.1212/01. WNL.0000147473.04043.B3.

Berkman, Lisa, and Lester Breslow. *Health and Ways of Living: The Alameda County Study*: New York: Oxford University Press, 1983.

Blanchflower, David, Andrew Oswald, and Sarah Stewart-Brown. "Is Psychological Wellbeing Linked to the Consumption of Fruit and Vegetables?" *Social Indicators Research* 114, no. 3 (2012): 785-801. https://doi.org/10.1007/s11205-012-0173-y.

Buysse, Daniel J. "Sleep Health: Can We Define It? Does It Matter?" *Sleep*. 37, no. 1 (2014): 9-17. https://doi.org/10.5665/sleep.3298.

Chida, Yoichi, and Andrew Steptoe. "Positive Psychological Wellbeing and Mortality: a Qualitative Review of Perspective Observational Studies." *Psychosomatic Medicine* 70 (September 2008): 741-756. https://doi.org/10.1097/PSY.0b013e31818105ba.

Cohen, Sheldon, William J Doyle, and David P Skoner. "Social Ties and Susceptibility to the Common Cold." *Journal of the American Medical Association* 277 (1997): 1940-44. https://doi.org/10.1001/jama.1997.03540480040036.

Cooney, Gary M, Kerry Dawn, Carolyn A Greig, Debbie A Lawlor, Jane Rimer, Fiona R Waugh, Marion Mcmurdo, and Gillian W Mead. "Exercise for Depression." *Cochrane Database Systematic Reviews* 9 (2013). https://doi.org/10.1002/14651858.CD004366.pub6.

Czekierda, Katarzyna, Anna Banik, Crustal L Park, and Aleksandra Luszczynska. "Meaning in Life and Physical Health: Systemic Review and Meta-Analysis." *Health Psychology Review* 11, no. 4 (2017): 387-418. https://doi.org/10.1080/17437199.2017.1327325.

Czikszentmihalyi, Mihalyi. *Flow: The Psychology of Optimal Experience*. New York, NY: Harper and Row, 1990.

D'Acquisto, Fulvio, and Alice Hamilton. "Cardiovascular and Immunological Implications of Social Distancing in the Context or COVID-19." *Cardiovascular Research* 116, no. 10 (2020): e129-e131. https://doi.org/10.1093/cvr/cvaa167.

Degarege, Abraham, Zaeema Naveed, Josiane Kabayundo, and David Brett-Major. "Risk Factors for Severe Illness and Death in COVID-19: A Systematic Review and Meta-Analysis." *Medrxiv* (2020). https://doi.org/10.1101/2020.12.03.20243659.

Emmons, Robert A, and Michael E. McCullough. "Counting Blessings Versus Burdens: Experimental Studies of Gratitude and Subjective Wellbeing." *Journal of Personality and Social Psychology* 84, no, 2 (2003): 377-389. https://doi.org/10.1037/0022-3514.84.2.377.

Frates, Beth, Jonathan P Bonnet, Richard Joseph, and James A Peterson. *Lifestyle Medicine Handbook, An Introduction to the Power of Health Habits*. Monterey, CA: Healthy Living, 2019.

Gardner, Meryl P, Briam Wansink, Junyong Kim, and Se-Bum Park. "Better Moods for Better Eating? How Mood Influences Food Choice." *Journal of Consumer Psychology* 24, no. 3 (2014): 320-335. https://doi.org/10.1016/j.jcps.2014.01.002.

Greater Good in Action, Science Practices for a Meaningful Life. University of California Berkeley: The Greater Good Science Center. https://ggia.berkeley.edu.

Harvard Study on Adult Development. https://www.adultdevelopmentstudy.org. Accessed June 23, 2021.

Hendriks, Ton, Marijke Schotanus-Dijkstra, Aabidien Hassankhan, Joop de Jong, and Ernst Bohlmeijer. "The Efficacy of Multi-component Positive Psychology Interventions: A Systematic Review and Meta-Analysis of Randomized Controlled Trials." *Journal of Happiness Studies* 21 (2020): 357-390. https://doi.org/10.1007/s10902-019-00082-1.

House, JS. "Social Isolation Kills, But How and Why?" *Psychosomatic Medicine* 63, (March/April 2001): 273-74. https://doi.org/10.1097/00006842-200103000-00011.

Kamerow, Douglas. "The Leading Cause of Death in the US." *British Medical Journal* 370 (August 2020): m3079. https://doi.org/10.1136/bmj.m3079.

Kim, Eric S, Victor J Strecher, and Carol Ryff. "Purpose in Life and Use of Preventive Health Care Services." *Proceedings in the National Academy of Sciences* 111, no. 46 (2014): 16331-16336. https://doi.org/10.1073/pnas.1414826111.

Kok, Bethany E, Kimberly A Coffey, Michael A Cohn, Lahnna I Catalino, Tanya Vacharklksemusk, Sara B Algoe, Mary Brantley, and Barbara Fredrickson. "How Positive Emotions Build Physical Health: Perceived Positive Social Connections Account for the Upward Spiral Between positive emotions and vagal tone." *Psychological Science* 24 (2013): 1123-1132. https://doi.org/10.1177/0956797612470827.

Lam, Raymond W, Anthony J Levitt, Robert D Levitan, Erin E Michalak, Amy H Cheung, R Morehouse R, Rajamannar Ramasubbu, Lakshmi N Yatham, and Edwin M Tam. "Efficacy of Bright Light Treatment, Fluoxetine, and the Combination in Patients with Nonseasonal Major Depressive Disorder: A Randomized Clinical Trial." *Journal of the American Medical Association Psychiatry* 23, no. 1 (2016): 56-63. https://doi.org/10.1001/jamapsychiatry.2015.2235.

Layous, Kristin, Huyunjung Lee, Incheol Choi, and Sonja Lyubomirsky. "Culture Matters When Designing a Successful Happiness-Increasing Activity: A Comparison of the United States and South Korea." *Journal of Cross-Cultural Psychology* 44 no. 8 (2013): 1294-1303. https://doi.org/10.1177/0022022113487591.

McGinnis JM and WH Foege. "Actual Causes of Death in the United States." *Journal of the American Medical Association* 270 (1993): 2207-2212. https://pubmed.ncbi.nlm.nih.gov/8411606.

Mujcic, Redzo, and Andrew J Oswald. "Evolution of Wellbeing and Happiness After Increases in Consumption of Fruit and Vegetables." *American Journal of Public Health.* 106, no. 8 (2016): 1504-10. https://doi.org/10.2105/AJPH.2016.303260.

Neff, Kristen. *Self-Compassion: The Proven Power of Being Kind to Yourself.* New York, NY: William Morrow Paperbacks, 2015.

Nelson-Coffey, S. Katherine, Megan M Fritz, Sonja Lyubomirsky, and Steve W Cole. "Kindness in the Blood: A Randomized Controlled Trial of the Gene Regulatory Impact of Prosocial Behavior." *Psychoneuroendocrinology* 81 (2017): 8-13. https://doi.org/10.1016/j.psyneuen.2017.03.025.

Ornish, Dean. *Love and Survival. 8 Pathways to Intimacy and Health.* New York, NY: Harper Perennial, HarperCollins Publishers, 1998.

Orth-Gomér, K, A Rosengren, and L Wilhelmsen. "Lack of Social Support and Incidence of Coronary Artery Disease in Middle-Aged Swedish Men." *Psychosomatic Medicine* 55 (January/February 1993): 37-43. https://doi.org/10.1097/00006842-199301000-00007.

Ozbay, Faith, Douglas C Johnson, Eleni Dimoulas, CA Morgan C A, Dennis Chamey, and Steven Southwick, "Social Support and Resilience to Stress." *Neurobiological Clinical Practice, Psychiatry (Edgemont)* 4, no. 5 (May 2007): 35-40.

Richards, Justin, Xiaoxiao Jiang, Paul Kelly, Josephine Chau, Adrian Bauman, and Ding Ding. Don't Worry, Be Happy: Cross-Sectional Associations Between Physical Activity and Happiness in 15 European Countries. *BMC Public Health* 15 (2015): article 53. https://www.ncbi.nlm.nih.gov/pmc/articles/PMC2921311.

Riopel, Leslie. The Importance, Benefits and Value of Goal Setting. October 4, 2019. Accessed June 23, 2021. https://positivepsychology.com/benefits-goal-setting.

Sandstrom, Gillian M, and Elizabeth W. Dunn. "Social Interactions and Wellbeing: The Surprising Power of Weak Ties."

Personality and Social Psychology Bulletin 40(2014): 910-922. https://doi.org/10.1177/0146167214529799.

Seligman, Martin. *Flourish: A Visionary New Understanding of Happiness and Wellbeing.* New York, NY: Free Press, 2011.

Tomaka, Joe, Sharon Thompson, and Rebecca Palacios. "The Relation of Social Isolation, Loneliness, and Social Support to Disease Outcomes among the Elderly." *Journal of Aging and Health* 18 (2006): 359-84. https://doi.org/10.1177/0898264305280993.

Vaillant, George E. *Triumphs of Experience: The Men of the Harvard Grant Study,* Cambridge, MA: Belknap Press, An imprint of Harvard University Press. 2012.

Umberson, Debra. "Family Status and Health Behaviors: Social Control as a Dimension of Social Integration." *Journal of Health and Social Behavior* 28 (1987): 306-19. https://doi.org/10.2307/2136848.

Whitehouse. Ralph Fiennes on Success. 2014. Accessed June 24, 2021. https://whitehousegbma.wordpress.com/2014/08/07/ralph-fiennes-on-success.

World Health Organization. The Top 10 Causes of Death. December 9, 2020. Accessed June 17, 2021. https://www.who.int/news-room/fact-sheets/detail/the-top-10-causes-of-death.

Li, Yanping, An Pan, Dang D Wang, Xiaoran Liu, Klodian Dhana, Oscar H Franco, Stephen Kaptage, Emanuele Di Angelantonio, Meir Stampfer, Walter C Willett, and Frank B Hu. "Impact of Healthy Lifestyle Factors on Life Expectancies in the US population." *Circulation* 138 (2018): 345-355. https://doi.org/10.1161/CIRCULATIONAHA.117.032047.

Chapter 4: Natural Strengths

Dweck, Carol S. *Mindset, The New Psychology of Success. How We Can Learn to Fulfill Our Potential.* New York City, NY: Ballantine Books, 2007.

Gardner, William L, and Mark J Martinko. "Using the Myers-Briggs Type Indicator to Study Managers: A Literature Review and Research Agenda." *Journal of Management.* 22, no. 1 (February 1996): 45-83. https://doi.org/10.1177/014920639602200103.

Lianov, Liana. *My Happy Avatar, Use Our Mobile Devise and Personality to Transform Your Health.* Fair Oaks, CA: HealthType LLC, 2013.

Myers, Isabella Briggs, and Peter B Myers. *Gifts Differing.* Palo Alto, CA: Consulting Psychologists Press, 1980.

Nardi, Dario. *Neuroscience of Personality, Brain Savvy Insights for All Types of People.* Los Angeles, CA: Radiance House, 2011.

Nardi, Dario. *The Magic Diamond, Jung's 8 Paths for Self-Coaching.* Los Angeles, CA: Radiance House, 2020.

Niemiec, Ryan M and Robert E McGrath. *The Power of Character Strengths, Appreciate and Ignite Your Positive Personality.* Cincinnati, Ohio: The Institute on Character, 2019.

Pittenger, David. Measuring the MBTI... and Coming Up Short. Marshall University. January 1993. https://www.researchgate.net/publication/237675975_Measurng_the_MBTI_and_coming_up_short.

Sharp, Daryl. *Personality Types, Jung's Model of Typology.* Toronto, Canada: Inner City Books, 1987.

The Myers & Briggs Foundation—The 16 MBTI® Types. Accessed June 26, 2012. https://www.myersbriggs.org/my-mbti-personality-type/mbti-basics/the-16-mbti-types.htm.

Virtues in Action Institute on Character. Accessed June 23, 2021. https://viacharacter.org/.

Chapter 5: Self-Care Strengths

Bratman, Gregory N, Gretchen C Daily, Benjamin J Levy, and James J Gross. "Benefits of Nature Experience: Improved Affect and Cognition." *Landscape and Urban Planning* 138 (2015): 41-50. https://doi.org/10.1016/j.landurbplan.2015.02.005.

Deci, Edward L. *Why We Do What We Do. Understanding Self-Motivation.* New York, NY: Penguin Books, 1995.

Jonas, Wayne. "Self-care: What Patients Want vs. What Physicians Can Provide." *AAFP News*, December 3, 2019. Accessed June 23, 2021. https://www.drwaynejonas.com/self-care-survey-2019.

Minich, Deanna. "A Review of the Science of Colorful, Plant-Based Food and Practical Strategies for 'Eating the Rainbow.'" *Journal of Nutrition and Metabolism* 2 (2019): 1-19. https://doi.org/10.1155/2019/2125070.

Twohig-Bennett, Caohime, and Andy Jones. "Health Benefits of the Great outdoors: A Systematic Review and Meta-Analysis of Greenspace Exposure and Health Outcomes." *Environmental Research* 166 (2018): 628-637. https://doi.org/10.1016/j.envres.2018.06.030.

Chapter 6: Positive Activity Strengths

Emmons, Robert A, and Michael E. McCullough. "Counting Blessings Versus Burdens: Experimental Studies of Gratitude and Subjective Wellbeing." *Journal of Personality and Social Psychology* 84, no, 2 (2003): 377-389. https://doi.org/10.1037/0022-3514.84.2.377.

Hendriks, Ton, Marijke Schotanus-Dijkstra, Aabidien Hassankhan, Joop de Jong, and Ernst Bohlmeijer. "The efficacy of multi-component Positive Psychology Interventions: A systematic review and meta-analysis of Randomized Controlled Trials." *Journal of Happiness Studies* 21 (2020): 357-390. https://doi.org/10.1007/s10902-019-00082-1.

Kabat-Zinn, John. "An Outpatient Program in Behavioral Medicine for Chronic Pain Patients Based on the Practice of Mindfulness Meditation: Theoretical Considerations and Preliminary Results." *General Hospital Psychiatry* 4, no. 1 (1982): 33-47. https://doi.org/10.1016/0163-8343(82)90026-3.

Koenig, Harold G. "Religion, Spirituality, and Health: The Research and Clinical Implications." *ISRN Psychiatry* (December 2020): 278730. https://doi.org/10.5402/2012/278730.

Kok, Bethany E, Kimberly A Coffey, Michael A Cohn, Lahnna I Catalino, Tanya Vacharklksemusk, Sara B Algoe, Mary Brantley, and Barbara Fredrickson. "How Positive Emotions Build Physical Health: Perceived Positive Social Connections Account for the Upward Spiral Between Positive Emotions and Vagal Tone." *Psychological Science* 24 (2013): 1123-1132. https://doi.org/10.1177/0956797612470827.

Layous, Kristin, Kennon M Sheldon, and Sonja Lyubomirsky. "The Prospects, Practices, and Prescription for the Pursuit of Happiness." In *Positive Psychology in Practice, Promoting Human Flourishing, in Work, Health, Education and Everyday Life* edited by Stephen Joseph. Hoboken, NJ: Wily, 2015.

Lustyk, M Kathleen B, Neharika Chawla, Roger Nolan, and G Alan Marlatt. "Mindfulness Meditation Research: Issues of Participant Screening, Safety Procedures, and Researcher Training." *Advances in Mind Body Medicine* 24, no. 1 (2009): 20-30. https://pubmed.ncbi.nlm.nih.gov/20671334/.

Michl, Louisa C, Katie A McLaughlin, Katherine Shepherd, and Susan Nolen-Hoeckesma. "Rumination as a Mechanism Linking Stressful Life Events to Symptoms of Depression and anxiety: Longitudinal Evidence in Early Adolescents and Adults."

Journal of Abnormal Psychology 122, no. 2 (2014): 339-352. https://doi.org/10.1037/a0031994.

Neff, Kristin, Kristin L Kirkpatrick, and Stephanie S Rude. "Self-Compassion and Adaptive Psychological Functioning." *Journal of Research in Personality* 41 (2007): 139-154. https://doi.org/10.1016/j.jrp.2006.03.004.

Niemiec, Ryan M, and Robert E McGrath. *The Power of Character Strengths, Appreciate and Ignite Your Positive Personality.* Cincinnati, Ohio: The Institute on Character, 2019.

Pressman, Sara D, and Sheldon Cohen. "Does Positive Affect Influence Health?" *Psychological Bulletin* 131, no. 6 (2005): 925-971. https://doi.org/10.1037/0033-2909.131.6.925.

Ryff, Carol. "Eudaimonic Wellbeing, Inequality, and Health: Recent Findings and Future Directions." *International Review of Economics* 64, no. 2 (2018): 159-178. https://doi.org/10.1007/s12232-017-0277-4.

Seligman, Martin. *Flourish: A Visionary New Understanding of Happiness and Wellbeing.* New York, NY: Free Press, 2011.

Steger, Michael F. "Meaning and wellbeing." In *Handbook of Wellbeing* edited by Edward Diener, Shigchiro, Oishi, and Louis Tay. Salt Lake City, UT: DEF Publishers, 2018.

Twohig-Bennett, Caohime, and Andy Jones. "Health Benefits of the Great Outdoors: A Systematic Review and Meta-Analysis of Greenspace Exposure and Health Outcomes." *Environmental Research* 166 (2018): 628-637. https://doi.org/10.1016/j.envres.2018.06.030.

Chapter 7: Social Connection Strengths

Algoe, Sara B. "Positive Interpersonal Processes." *Current Directions in Psychological Science* 28, no. 2 (2019);183-188.

https://doi.org/10.1177/0963721419827272.

Algoe, Sara B, Patrick C Dwyer, Ayana Younge, and Christopher Oveis. "A New Perspective on the Social Functions of Emotions: Gratitude and the Witnessing Effect." *Journal of Personality and Social Psychology* 119, no. 1 (2019): 40-74. https://doi.org/10.1037/pspi0000202.

American Psychological Association. "Stress in America™ 2020, A National Mental Health Crisis." Accessed June 23, 2021. https://www.apa.org/news/press/releases/stress/2020/report-october.

Brailovskaia Julia, and Jürgen Margraf. "Facebook Addiction Disorder (FAD) among German students—A Longitudinal Approach." *PLoS ONE* 12, no. 12 (2017): e0189719. https://doi.org/10.1371/journal.pone.0189719.

Dutton, James E, and Emily D Heaphy. "The Power of High-Quality Connections." In *Positive Organizational Scholarship* edited by Kim Cameron Jane E Dutton, and Robert Quinn, 2003, p. 263-278.

Frates Beth, Jonathan P, Richard Joseph R, James A Peterson. *Lifestyle Medicine Handbook, An Introduction to the Power of Healthy Habits.* Monterey, CA: Healthy Living, 2019, p. 342-346.

Gable, Shelly L, and Emily A Impett. "Approach and Avoidance Motives and Close Relationships." *Social and Personality Psychology Compass* 6, no. 1 (2012): 95-108. https://doi.org/10.1111/j.1751-9004.2011.00405.x.

Johnson, Julienne K, Anita L Stewart, Michael Acree, Anna M Nápoles, Jason D Flatt, Wendy B Max, and Steven E Gregorich. "A Community Choir Intervention to Promote Wellbeing Among Diverse Older Adults: Results from the Community of Voices Trial." *The Journals of Gerontology: Series B.* 75, no. 3 (2020): 549-559. https://doi.org/10.1093/geronb/gby132.

Kemp S. We Are Social. *Digital 2020: 3.8 Billion People Use Social Media*. January 30, 2020. Accessed June 24, 2021. https://wearesocial.com/blog/2020/01/digital-2020-3-8-billion-people-use-social-media.

Knapp, Mark L, Judith A Hall, and Terrance G Horgan. *Nonverbal Communication in Human Interaction* (8th edition). Boston, MA: Cengage Learning, 2013.

Kok, Bethany E, Kimberly A Coffey, Michael A Cohn, Lahnna I Catalino, Lahnna I, Tanya Vacharklksemusk, Sara B Algoe, Mary Brantley, and Barbara Fredrickson. "How Positive Emotions Build Physical Health: Perceived Positive Social Connections Account for the Upward Spiral Between Positive Emotions and Vagal Tone." *Psychological Science* 24(2013): 1123-1132. https://doi.org/10.1177/0956797612470827.

Kurtz LE and Sara B Algoe. "When Sharing a Laugh Means Sharing More: Testing the Role of Shared Laughter on Short-Term Interpersonal Consequences. *Journal of Nonverbal Behavior* 41, no. 1 (2017): 45-65. https://doi.org/10.1007/s10919-016-0245-9.

Lin, Liu yi, Jaime E Sidani, Ariel Shensa, Ana Radovic, Elizabeth Miller, Jason B Colditz, Beth L Hoffman, Leila M Giles, and Brian A Primack. "Association Between Social Media Use and Depression Among US Young Adults." *Depression and Anxiety* 33, no. 4 (2016): 323-331. https://doi.org/10.1002/da.22466.

Martino, Jessica, Jennifer Pegg, and Elizabeth Pegg Frates. "The Connection Prescription: Using the Power of Social Interactions and the Deep Desire for Connectedness to Empower Health and Wellness." *American Journal of Lifestyle Medicine* 11, no. 6(2017): 466-475. https://doi.org/10.1177/1559827615608788.

Ornish, Dean. Presentation at the virtual Lifestyle Medicine 2020 conference, American College of Lifestyle Medicine, October 22, 2020.

Ornish, Dean. *Love and Survival. 8 Pathways to Intimacy and Health.* New York, NY: Harper Perennial, HarperCollins Publishers, 1998.

Sandstrom, Gillian M, and Elizabeth W. Dunn. "Social Interactions and Wellbeing: The Surprising Power of Weak Ties." *Personality and Social Psychology Bulletin* 40 (2014): 910-922. https://doi.org/10.1177/0146167214529799.

Seabrook, Elizabeth M, Margaret L Kern, and Nikki S Rickard. "Social Networking Sites, Depression, and Anxiety: A Systemic Review." *JMIR Mental Health* 3, no. 4 (October—November 2016): e50. https://www.doi.org/10.2196/mental.5842.

Umerson, Debra, and Jennifer Karas Montez. "Social Relationships and Health: A Flashpoint for Health Policy." *Journal of Health and Social Behavior* 51 (2010): S54-S66. https://doi.org/10.1177/0022146510383501.

Vaillant, George E. *Triumphs of Experience: The Men of the Harvard Grant Study.* Cambridge, MA: Belknap Press, An imprint of Harvard University Press, 2012

Vannucci, Anna, Kaitlin M Flannery, and Christine McCauley Ohannessian. "Social Media Use and Anxiety in Emerging Adults." *Journal of Affective Disorders* 207 (2017): 163-166. https://doi.org/10.1016/j.jad.2016.08.040.

Waters, Lea, Sara B Algoe, Jane Dutton, Robert Emmons, Barbara L Fredrickson, Emily Heaphy, Judith T Moskowitz, Kristin Neff, Ryan Niemiec, Cynthia Pury, and Michael Steger. "Positive Psychology in a Pandemic: Buffering, Bolstering, and Building Mental Health." *The Journal of Positive Psychology.* February 9, 2021. https://doi.org/10.1080/17439760.2021.1871945.

Chapter 8: Character Strengths

Kaufman, Scott Barry. "Which Character Strengths Are Most Predictive of Wellbeing." *Scientific American*. August 2, 2015. https://blogs.scientificamerican.com/beautiful-minds/which-character-strengths-are-most-predictive-of-well-being.

Niemiec, Ryan M and Richard E McGrath. *The Power of Character Strengths. Official Guide from the VIA Institute on Character.* VIA Institute on Character, 2019.

Sheldon, Kennon M, Paul E Jose, Todd B Kashdan, and Aaron Jarden. "Personality, Effective Striving, and Enhanced Wellbeing: Comparing 10 Candidate Personality Strengths." *Personality and Social Psychology Bulletin* 41, no. 4 (February 2015): 575-585. https://doi.org/10.1177/0146167215573211.

VIA Institute on Character. Accessed June 23, 2021. https://www.viacharacter.org.

Chapter 9: Brain Strengths

Lianov, Liana. *My Happy Avatar, Use Our Mobile Devise and Personality to Transform Your Health.* Fair Oaks, CA: HealthType LLC, 2013.

Myers Isabella Briggs and Peter Briggs Myers. *Gifts Differing.* Palo Alto, CA: Consulting Psychologists Press, 1980.

Nardi, Dario. *Neuroscience of Personality, Brain Savvy Insights for All Types of People.* Los Angeles, CA: Radiance House, 2011.

Nardi, Dario. *The Magic Diamond, Jun's 8 Paths for Self-Coaching.* Los Angeles, CA: Radiance House, 2020.

Quenk, Naomi. *Was That Really Me? How Everyday Stress Brings Out Our Hidden Personality.* Boston, MA: Nicholas Brealey, 2002.

The Myers & Briggs Foundation. Accessed June 26, 2021. https://www.myersbriggs.org.

Chapter 10: Reliable Strengths during Traumatic Times

Niemiec, Ryan M and Richard McGrath. *The Power of Character Strengths, Appreciate and Ignite Your Positive Personality*. VIA Institute in Character, 2019.

Chapter 11: Strengths in Action

Aghera, Amish, Matt Emery, Richard Bounds, Colleen Bush, R Brent Stansfield, Brian Gillett, and Sally A Santen, Sally A. "A Randomized Trial of SMART Goal Enhanced Debriefing After Simulation to Promote Educational Actions." *West Journal of Emergency Medicine* 19, no. 1 (2018): 112-120. https://doi.org/10.5811/westjem.2017.11.36524.

Claiborn, James and Cherry Pedrick. *The Habit Change Workbook, How to Break Bad Habits and Form Good Ones*. Oakland, CA: New Harbinger Publications, Inc., 2001.

Education Planner. What's Your Learning Style? The Learning Styles. Accessed June 10, 2021. http://www.educationplanner.org/students/self-assessments/learning-styles-styles.shtml.

Fogg, B J. *Tiny Habits, The Small Changes that Change Everything*. Boston, MA: Houghton Mifflin Harcourt USA, 2019.

Kok, Bethany E, Kimberly A Coffey, Michael A Cohn, Lahnna I Catalino, Tanya Vacharklksemusk, Sara B Algoe, Mary Brantley, and Barbara Fredrickson. "How Positive Emotions Build Physical Health: Perceived Positive Social Connections Account for the Upward Spiral Between Positive Emotions and

Vagal Tone." *Psychological Science* 24 (2013): 1123-1132. https://doi.org/10.1177/0956797612470827.

Moore, Margaret, and Bob Tschannen-Moran. *Coaching Psychology Manual*. Philadelphia, Pennsylvania: Walters Kluwer, Lippincott Williams & Wilkins, 2010.

The National Board of Health and Wellness Coaching website. Accessed June 24, 2021. https://nbhwc.org.

Rollnick, Stephen, Pip Mason, and Chris Butler. *Health Behavior Change, A Guide for Practitioners*. New York, NY: Churchill Livingstone, 2002.

Watson, Stephanie. Relapse Prevention Plan: Techniques to Help You Stay on Track. January 7, 2020. Accessed June 23, 2021. https://healthline.com/health/opioid-withdrawal/relapse-prevention-plan.

Resources: Identifying Brain Strengths

Kroeger, Otto and Janet M, Thuesen. *Type Talk, The 16 Personality Types That Determine How We Live, Love and Work*. New York City, NY: Dell Publishing, 1989.

Lianov, Liana. *My Happy Avatar, Use Our Mobile Devise and Personality to Transform Your Health*. Fair Oaks, CA: HealthType LLC, 2013.

Acknowledgements

Dr. Seuss. *Did I Ever Tell You How Lucky You Are?* New York, NY: Random House Books for Young Readers, 1973.

Made in United States
Orlando, FL
18 January 2025